THE HEARTBREAK OF

ALZHEIMER'S

by

Mabel V. Pollock

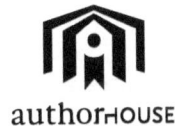

authorHOUSE

1663 LIBERTY DRIVE, SUITE 200
BLOOMINGTON, INDIANA 47403
(800) 839-8640
www.authorhouse.com

First published by AuthorHouse 05/04/04

ISBN: 1-4184-0052-1 (e)
ISBN: 1-4184-0053-X (sc)

Library of Congress Control Number: 2004091654

Printed in the United States of America
Bloomington, Indiana

This book is printed on acid-free paper.

This is a true, first-hand account of how Alzheimer's disease affected a victim, his family and friends. It was written by his wife, the principle caregiver.

FOREWORD

Alzheimer's is a disease which affects an estimated four million American adults. It ranks fourth as the cause of death in persons over 75 years of age. Approximately 6% of persons 65 to 75 years of age, 10% of those 75 to 85 years of age, and 20% of those over 85 suffer from it. Approximately 1% to 10% of its victims develop symptoms in their fifties, forties, or even their thirties.

Alzheimer's is a brain disorder in which nerve cells in memory areas of the brain and, eventually, other areas begin to die at an accelerated rate. It usually involves progressive memory loss, but difficulties with vision, speech and emotions are also common. Deterioration in cognitive skills may continue for five to ten years.

Alzheimer's disease was first recognized in a fifty-one year old woman in the early 1900's by Alois Alzheimer, a physician in Frankfurt-am-Main, Germany.

At the onset, personality changes are so subtle that even those persons closest to him, or her, are often not aware that there is a problem. As the disease progresses, bad judgment, forgetfulness and confusion become obvious. Family members and friends are often bewildered by these changes.

Medications have been developed which slow the progress of the disease, but there is no known cure for it at this time.

My husband, Ralph's condition was diagnosed as Alzheimer's in 1996 and since I had worked as a newspaper reporter, I was accustomed to jotting down notes. From my memory and these notes, I have compiled the following book which is a true account of the progress of this devastating disease and how it affected Ralph, his family and friends.

Mabel V. Pollock

TABLE OF CONTENTS

CHAPTER I

HIS BACKGROUND

Ralph Pollock was born in Akron, Ohio on January 1, 1921. He grew up on a farm near Newcomerstown. He graduated from the local high school in 1938 and took a job at the local Heller Brothers Tool Company. In 1942, six months after the Japanese attack on Pearl Harbor, he was inducted into the U.S. Army. Following basic training, he was assigned to a Machine Records Unit and stationed in New Orleans, Louisiana. In February, 1943, he came home on furlough and we were married. I accompanied him back to New Orleans, but he was soon assigned to overseas duty and I returned home. Ralph spent the next three and one-half years in the Bismarck Archipelago, New Guinea, The Philippines, Luzon and Japan. He was promoted to the rank of T-4 Sergeant and earned the WWII Victory Medal; The American Theatre

Ribbon; The Asiatic-Pacific Theatre Ribbon with 4 bronze stars; The Philippine Liberation Ribbon with 1 bronze star, and the Good Conduct Ribbon.

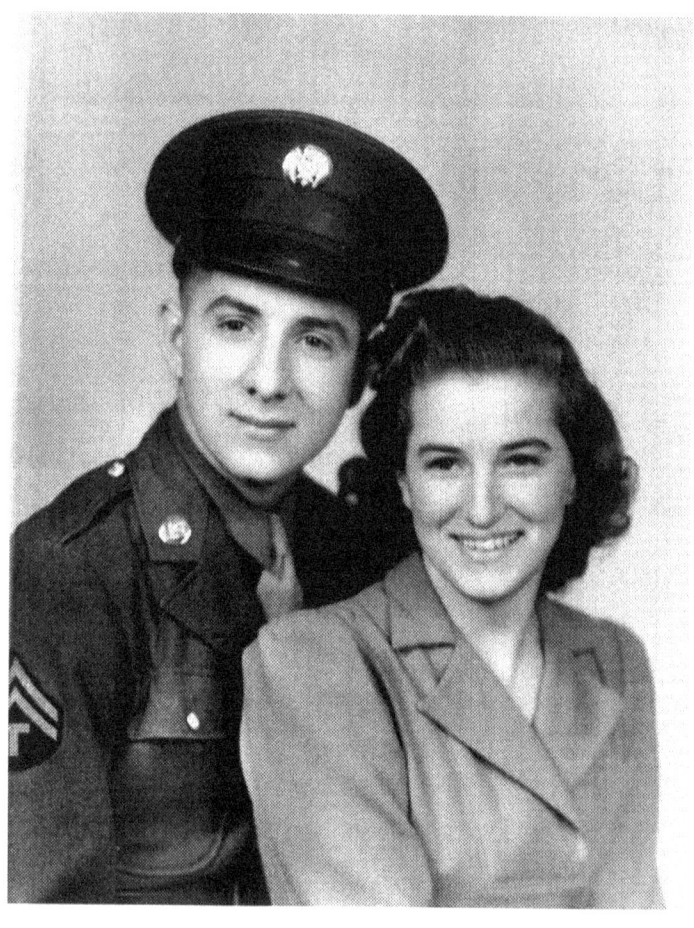

Ralph Pollock and Mabel Hayes were married on February 11, 1943 while he was home on furlough.

He was on a ship with the Sixth Army which was on the way to participate in the invasion of Japan when, on August 6, 1945, the atomic bomb was dropped on Hiroshima. Two days later, on August 8, another atomic bomb was dropped on Nagasaki. The war was soon over and there is no doubt in my mind that the use of those bombs saved many American lives, including my husband's, and many Japanese lives as well.

Casualties among invasion forces had been estimated at such a high level that the U.S. Army had stockpiled a large supply of coffins and body bags to ship bodies back to the U.S.

Ralph returned home safely in January, 1946. He never seemed to want to discuss his military service, but he was especially proud that he had served his country.

Ralph resumed his job at the local tool company and we rented a house in town. That fall, we purchased a 30-acre farm near Shadybend, about a mile west of Newcomerstown, using the money we had saved while he was in the army.

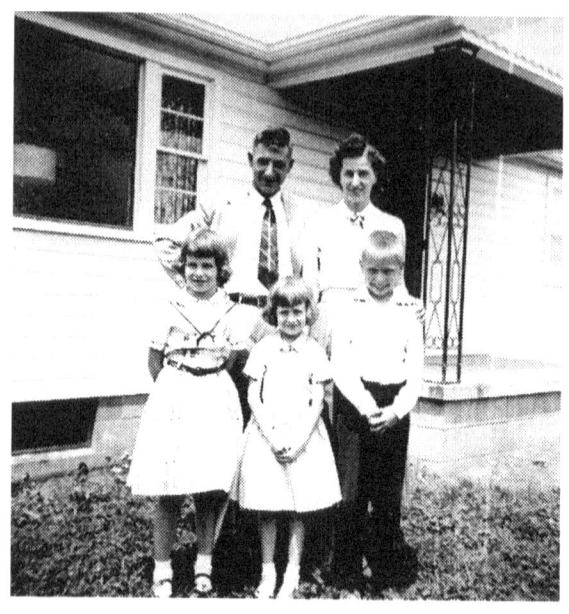

The Ralph L. Pollock Family in 1956: Ralph, Mabel, Janet, Karen, Dennis.

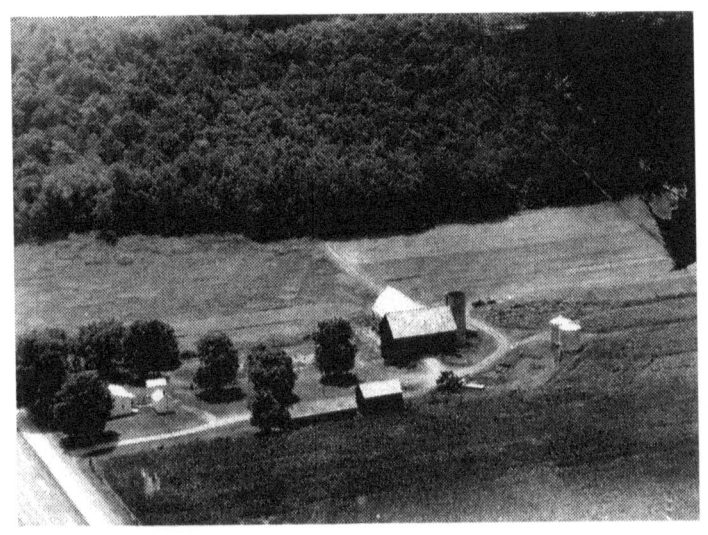

We purchased this farm in 1952. It is located in Oxford Township, Coshocton County..

Our first child, Dennis, was born in November, 1946; Janet, in July, 1948; and Karen, in November, 1949.

Ralph had always wanted to be a farmer, and, in 1952, we sold the farm in Shadybend and purchased the 231 acre farm where I reside.

Ralph worked hard on the farm and, although farm income was often below the average income of other segments of the economy, we managed to pay off the mortgage and financed our daughter's college education.

CLOUDS OF WAR

During the 1960's, the clouds of war once again cast an ominous shadow over our lives. In 1966, when it became apparent that Dennis, our only son, would be drafted, he chose to enlist in the U.S. Navy Seabees, a construction unit.

In March of 1967, while stationed at Camp LeJeune, North Carolina to train for duty in Vietnam, he went swimming. He was a good swimmer and had taken the Red Cross Lifesaving course. However, he was unfamiliar with the tides which raise and lower the water level and he dove into shallow water, fractured his neck and died from the injury.

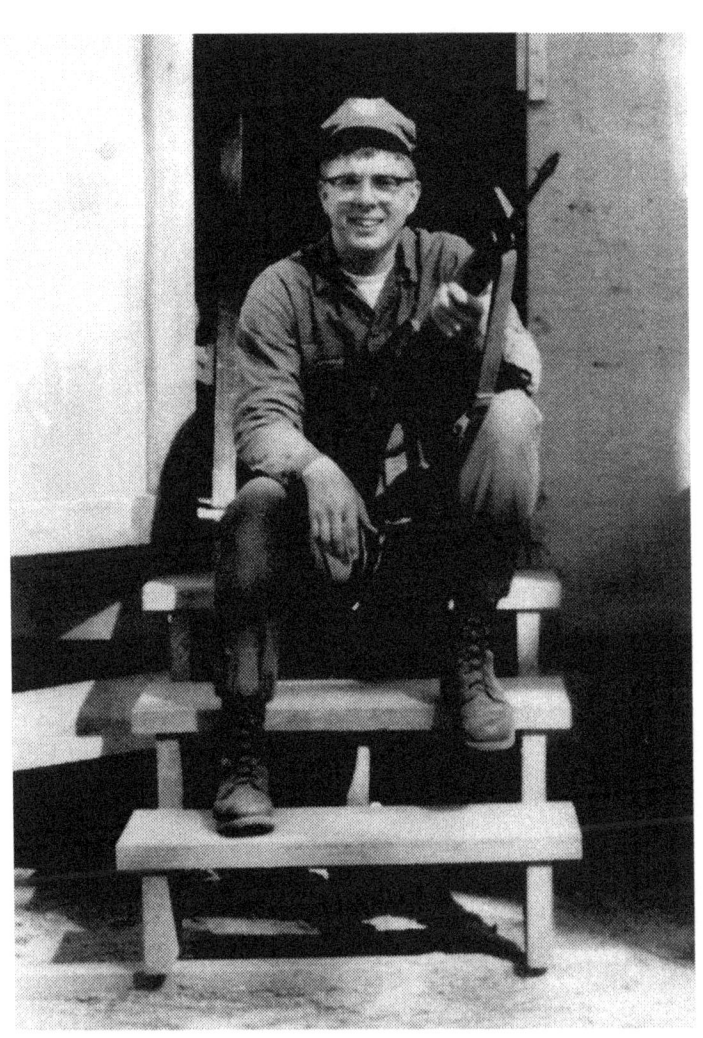

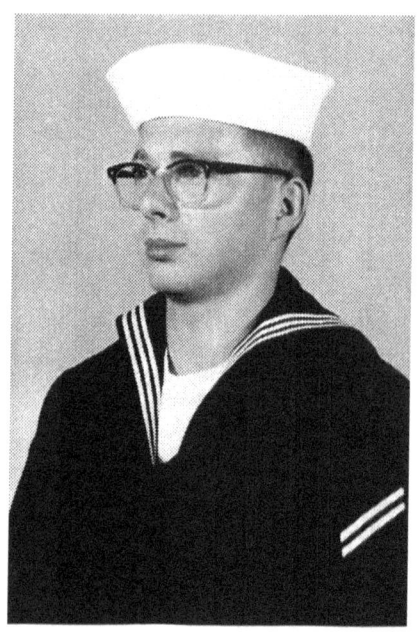

Seaman First Class, U.S. Navy Seabees.
Dennis Lynn Pollock, our only son, who died in a swimming accident
while stationed at Camp LeJeune, North Carolina to train for duty in
Vietnam.

Although Ralph seldom allowed his true feelings to show, I don't believe he ever recovered from the shock of our tragic loss and, neither did our daughters and I. But, life goes on. We became more appreciative of our daughters and our loss drew us all closer together.

I resigned my job to spend more time with my daughters before they went away to college that fall.

CHAPTER II

HEALTH PROBLEMS

Ralph's health problems began in 1987. We had been in Florida visiting Karen and her family. We returned home early in February because we planned to travel to Wisconsin for the birth of our youngest grandchild. We had been home for only two days when, on a cold, February morning, Ralph complained of a pain in his left arm. I asked him if he thought it might be his heart and he said, "Yes."

I immediately got the car out and drove him to the Emergency Room of the Coshocton County Memorial Hospital where his condition was confirmed as a heart attack. He was hospitalized for two weeks and started on the medications, Procardia and Inderol. We cancelled our trip to Wisconsin and did not get to meet our new baby granddaughter, Sara, until the middle of August when Janet and her family came to Ohio to attend a family reunion.

Ralph recovered completely from his heart attack and lived a normal life for the next six years. He rented out his cropland to ease the burden of farming, but continued to raise sweet corn which we sold at a roadside stand.

He also continued to make hay which we hauled to auctions at Farmerstown, Mount Hope and Kidron. He enjoyed fishing, playing cards, hunting deer, traveling to Wisconsin to visit Janet and her family, and to Florida to visit Karen and her family. There were no noticeable symptoms of Alzheimer's at this stage.

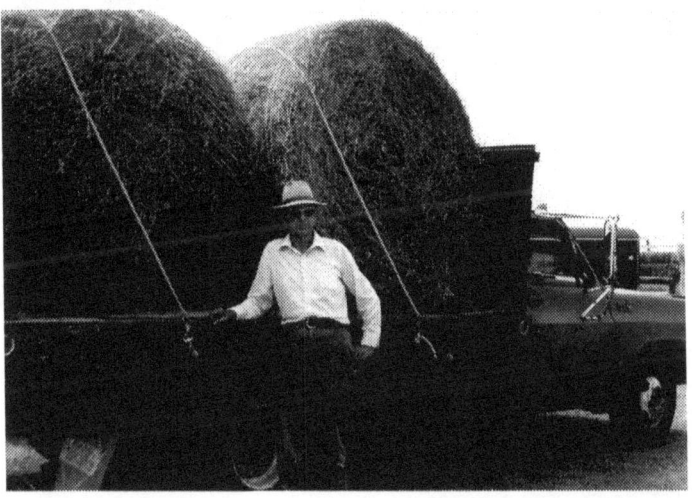

Ralph enjoyed making large, round bales of hay and hauling them to the hay auctions at Farmerstown, Mount Hope and Kidron.

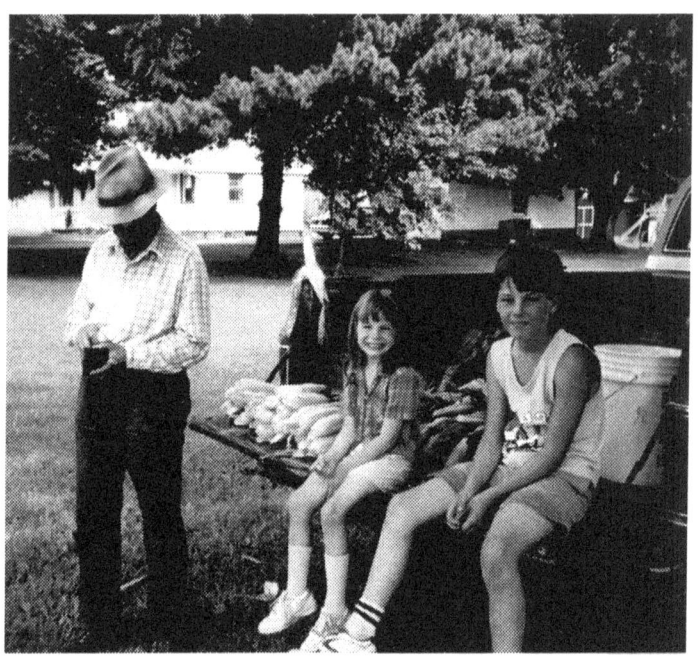

Ralph also enjoyed raising sweet corn which we sold at a roadside
stand. Our grandchildren, Ben and Sara, liked to help.

MORE HEALTH PROBLEMS

In April, 1993, Ralph began to have heart problems again. His physician referred him to Mount Carmel Medical Center at Columbus where he underwent angioplasty.

Two years later, on June 27, 1995, he was hospitalized at Southeastern Regional Medical Center, Cambridge where a small clot was found in his heart.

Two months later, from August 7 to August 13, he was again treated at Mount Carmel Medical Center for a stroke and heart condition. On October 3, he underwent cardiac catherization.

By November, his condition had stabilized and he seemed well enough to travel to Florida. His doctor had advised that he avoid extremely cold weather which seemed to aggravate his condition.

On November 27, two weeks after we arrived there, he was admitted to Florida Hospital Walker at Avon Park. It was then known as Walker Hospital. He was treated for a bleeding ulcer believed caused by taking Coumadin and aspirin together.

CHAPTER III

THE FIRST SYMPTOM

On November 30, I left the hospital about 5:30 p.m. and returned to our apartment which was about two miles away in Avon Park. About 6:30 p.m., the hospital called and informed me that my husband was not in his room and they had been unable to locate him. I called my daughter, Karen, and son-in-law, Larry, and they were soon on the way from Miami to Avon Park.

I also called Ralph's sister and her husband who were spending the winter near us and we rushed to the hospital immediately.

Two of the hospital's security guards were searching the hospital and grounds for him. We asked that they notify the sheriff's department and the Avon Park police because the hospital was located in Highlands County, but we lived in Avon Park. It was a frightening situation. There were several small lakes in the area and it was very dark outside. I feared that he might be attempting to walk to our apartment dressed in hospital pajamas and house slippers.

A sheriff's deputy arrived along with a tracking dog. The dog was allowed to sniff some of Ralph's clothing and soon picked up his trail.

Ralph was located about three hours later. He had pulled out his I.V., yanked his heart monitor off and threw it away, then walked along the railroad tracks to our apartment. When he found the door locked, he went to a neighbor's apartment. She recognized him and knew that he had been in the hospital. Although she was having a card party, she invited him into her kitchen, seated him on a chair and gave him a blanket to wrap up in. She then called the sheriff and Ralph was returned to the hospital, unharmed except for scratches on his ankles from walking through briars.

Soon after Ralph was safely back in his hospital bed, my daughter and son-in-law arrived and helped to calm me down.

Although I had begun to notice that Ralph often turned to me to answer questions or to identify people he formerly knew quite well, I had never been around anyone who had Alzheimer's disease and had always attributed his forgetfulness to his age. However, after he walked out of the hospital in his pajamas, I began to wonder if he had a problem, and I believe that that incident was the first noticeable sign that he had a problem, a serious problem. I made an appointment with a neurologist.

THE DIAGNOSIS

Ralph was dismissed from Florida Hospital Walker on December 1, 1995. His driving was still good and we drove to Miami from Avon Park to spend Christmas with our daughter, son-in-law and two granddaughters. We made several trips to the Auburndale flea market where we could purchase fresh produce. Ralph went fishing with his friends and we played cards often. He seemed normal in every respect except for his mild forgetfulness.

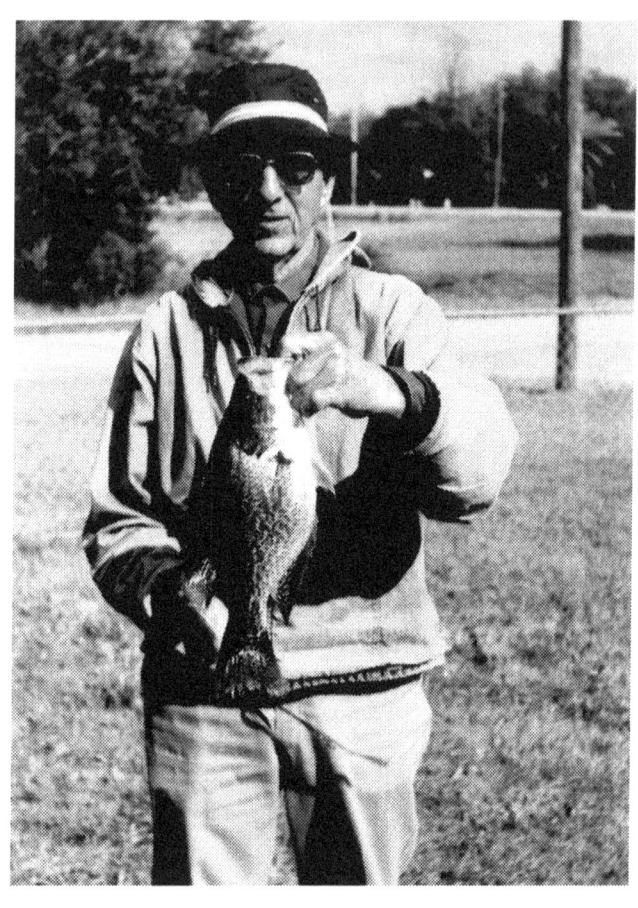

Ralph enjoyed fishing in Florida and the size of the crappie he caught explains why.

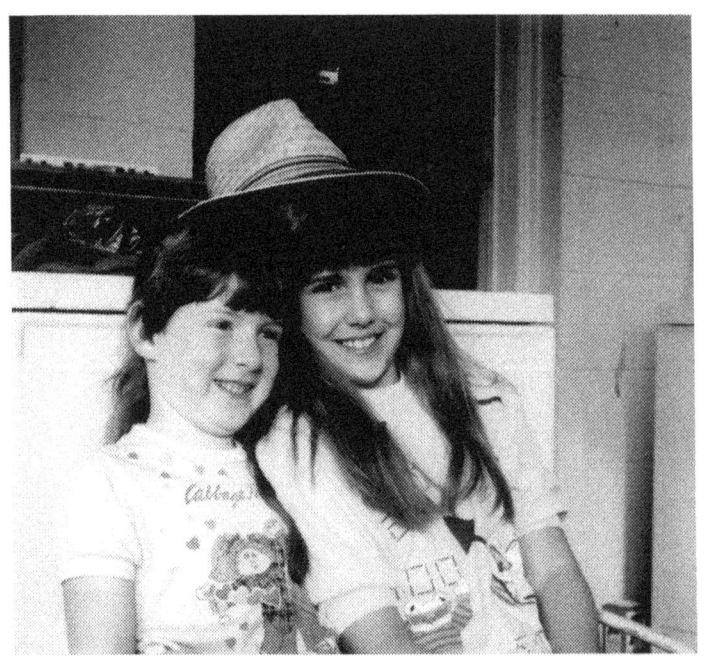

Our granddaughters, Christina and Cheryl, enjoyed wearing "Grandpa's fishing hat."

After Ralph recovered from his bleeding ulcer, we consulted Dr. Khara of the Sebring Neurological Center. Ralph was referred to a psychologist for extensive testing and his condition was diagnosed as Dementia of the Alzheimer's type. He was started on Cognex, the current medication for Alzheimer's at that time.

By March of 1996, Ralph's doctor determined that he was well enough to travel, and, we returned to Ohio.

CHAPTER IV

CONFUSION

By May of 1996, Ralph had become unable to farm as he formerly did and, subsequently, our income suffered. We needed money for expenses and decided to sell a parcel of land. We listed 68 acres of good, level bottom land which was underlaid with gravel, with an area real estate auctioneer. We specified that we wished to reserve the right to reject the last bid, but the auctioneer listed it in the newspaper ads as "Absolute Auction." We contacted a lawyer who consulted the auctioneer who then agreed to announce that we reserved the right to reject the last bid. The lawyer attended the sale to insure that it was handled properly.

A few weeks before the sale, I suspected that Ralph was having problems when he asked on at least two occasions, "Which piece of land are we selling?" I began to think that we should not go through with the sale, but, when I suggested that we cancel it, Ralph became quite upset.

Our daughter, Janet, was also concerned and she suggested to him that we postpone the sale; but, he became upset with her, too.

The land sold for $1,800 per acre, although similar land in the area had recently sold for $2,400 per acre.

FORGETFULNESS

By the beginning of 1997, Ralph's forgetfulness and confusion became quite apparent.

He parked his tractor on the barn bank and forgot to set the brake. The tractor rolled down the bank into the side of his long-bed hay truck, denting the door.

He added water to the gas tank of his tractor. Fortunately, a friend stopped by and helped him drain it.

He left the key to his tractor turned on and the battery ran down.

He placed a glove over the furnace pipe on the outside of the house, causing the furnace to malfunction. When I asked him why he did that, he explained, "My glove had gotten wet and I thought that would be a good place to dry it."

On day, as he sat in his favorite chair looking out the living room window, he said, "I wonder where that road goes."

"What road?" I asked.

"That road," he replied and pointed to the neighbor's driveway.

Early in 1998, Ralph's Neurologist discontinued the Cognex and started him on Aricept, the latest Alzheimer's medication at that time. But, sadly, his memory continued to fade.

He forgot how to operate some of his machinery. When he couldn't get his disc-bine to work, a neighbor borrowed it and it worked just fine.

He left the lights on in his truck and the battery ran down. He misplaced his keys, coat and hat and we spent hours searching for them. I believe he left them in a restaurant.

When he wanted to get a haircut, I accompanied him to town. He parked in front of the barbershop and when I noticed there were several others ahead of him, I told him that I would walk up the street to the bank. When I returned he had left without me and without getting his hair cut. I called a friend to take me home and when we got there, he was sitting on the back porch, smiling.

"Well," he said, "I wondered where you were." He was blissfully unaware that he had left me stranded in town. From then on, I kept all keys in my possession.

FLAWED JUDGMENT

When Ralph had difficulty getting his hay rake to work properly, he insisted on buying a used one from an area implement dealer. He paid $1,000 for it, but he had trouble getting it to work and I suspected he had forgotten how to operate much of his machinery.

Finally, he insisted on taking it back to the dealer, but the dealer said it was too late in the season to resell it at that time.

I asked them if they would be willing to hold it over and sell it at the beginning of the next hay season and they said they would try. However, several years later we have heard nothing from them and they still have the rake and our $1,000.

Other instances of questionable judgment included loaning a log splitter to an acquaintance who never returned it; and, selling hay bales to a party who never paid for some of them.

There were other incidents which I will not mention here.

Ralph was aware that he had Alzheimer's. His Neurologist had explained it to both of us in February, 1996, when it was diagnosed and Ralph seemed to understand what it meant.

I believed it was very important to keep him active as long as possible. However, I feared that he might be injured while trying to operate his haymaking equipment which was very dangerous. I suggested that we let someone else make the hay on the shares and we would continue to haul it to the hay auctions at Farmerstown, Mount Hope and Kidron in the pick-up truck, which I could operate, instead of the long-bed hay truck. To my surprise, he agreed to this. We rented out all cropland except for a plot on which to raise sweet corn which we sold at a roadside stand.

I believe that hauling hay to market and working with the sweet corn helped to keep his mind alert longer than it would have been if we had denied him these pleasures.

CHAPTER V

STILL MORE SYMPTOMS

As time went on, Ralph gradually became more and more dependent upon me. His driving became erratic and I began to accompany him everywhere. He had difficulty remembering where to turn off the highway and, occasionally, went through stoplights. Once, he lost his way while hauling hay to the hay auction.

One day in August, 1999, as we were on our way to the Farmer's Market at Coshocton to sell sweet corn, we stopped at a service station to check the water and oil in the pick-up truck. We also purchased some antifreeze and used part of it. I handed the jug to Ralph and asked him to put it in the back of the truck while I went inside to pay. When I came back out, he was trying to put the antifreeze in the gas tank. I got there just in time and I believe he thought I meant for him to put the antifreeze in the gas tank.

On August 26, 1999, I had begun to mow the lawn when Ralph came outside and wanted to help. I turned the garden tractor over to him and went inside the house. A short time later, I glanced out the kitchen window and noticed that smoke was coming from the garden tractor. I hurried outside and discovered that Ralph had one foot on the gas pedal and the other on the brake.

By October, Ralph was still well enough to travel and we decided to visit Janet in Wisconsin. We decided to travel by airplane since Ralph's driving was getting worse. We took a flight to Chicago where we changed planes to Minneapolis – St. Paul. In the terminal at O'Hare airport, we were on an escalator and Ralph was directly behind me. When we reached the second level, I got off and looked around, but Ralph was nowhere in sight. I ran alongside the horizontal moving sidewalk until I spied him. He had followed the flow of people onto the moving sidewalk. I intercepted him at the next exit and vowed that, the next time we would take a direct flight.

By November of 1999, Ralph seemed well enough to travel to Florida. We had many friends there and we enjoyed visiting the flea markets, especially the one at Auburndale where we could purchase fresh produce. But, most of all, we looked forward to visiting our daughter, Karen, and her family at Miami.

Ralph enjoyed fishing in Florida and usually went with a friend, but, when his friend was unavailable, I accompanied him. The last time we fished in Lake Placid, he became confused and couldn't remember where the boat ramp was located. I tried to point it out to him, but he went past it and had to turn around and come back. That would be the last fishing trip for us.

On our way home from Florida in March, 2000, Ralph became confused and thought we were on the wrong road. He wanted to stop at the next town and find out where we were. I was driving and told him that I knew the way home and we had to keep moving so we could get home before dark. We reached home shortly after dark. I unlocked the door and we went in. "How did you get in here?" he asked. "Who owns this place?"

That would be our last trip to Florida.

Each day it seemed that Ralph's confusion, forgetfulness and bad judgment became more obvious.

He often forgot to take his pills and, when I gave them to him, he would spit them out into the wastebasket.

I placed letters in the mailbox to be mailed out, but he brought them back into the house, thinking they were incoming mail.

He picked field corn, thinking it was sweet corn and wanted to sell it.

He couldn't remember what day of the week it was and wanted to haul hay to the hay auctions every day.

He had trouble remembering where the bathroom is and tried to wear socks for gloves.

CHAPTER VI

HE FORGOT HOW TO DRESS

The year 2000 was a stressful year for me. Ralph forgot how to dress; he forgot where he lived; and, at times he forgot that I was his wife.

A few times, he attempted to put his clothes on over his pajamas. He tried to put his legs into the sleeves of his shirt. Once, he came downstairs wearing my white, cotton slacks; and, at bedtime, he tried to wear his pajamas over his regular clothes. Once, he wore my blouse for a pajama top.

He tied his shoestrings in many knots and tried to wear his shoes to bed.

"Oh, why do you keep doing things like that?" I asked him as I untangled his shoestrings.

"I can't help it," he replied, calmly as a tear slid down his cheek.

I realized that he had reached a stage of the disease in which he couldn't control his actions; and, I vowed never to speak to him in that tone of voice again because, like many other Alzheimer's victims, he couldn't help doing the things he did.

HE FORGOT WHERE HE LIVED

By the fall of 2000, there were times when Ralph did not recognize our home. Almost every evening, he would say, "I'm ready to go home."

I would try to explain to him that we were already home. We had lived here for more than fifty years. When I couldn't convince him, I asked, "Where do you think your home is?"

"Shadybend," he replied.

Ralph had lived on a farm in Shadybend, about a mile north of our present home, from about the age of seven until he entered the U.S. Army. I believe that his mind had regressed back to his childhood.

I began to take him for a ride every evening. I would drive past the site of his childhood home and explain that the house he had lived in had burned down many years ago and had been replaced. Then, we would return to our home and he was usually satisfied. However, there were times when I had to take him for a second ride.

HE FORGOT HIS WIFE

As the disease continued to devastate his mind, he often forgot that I was his wife. He began to call me "Dorothy," which was his sister's name.

One day, he was in an especially good mood, and he said to me, "I'm going to marry you if I can find my license." However, a short time later, he had evidently changed his mind because he said, "No, I'm not going to marry you. You're too bossy."

At times he would ask me, "Where's Mabel? She was here a little while ago."

When I couldn't convince him that I was Mabel, I would call a family member who would try to convince him that I was, indeed, his wife, Mabel.

HE FORGOT THAT THE CHILDREN HAD LEFT HOME

As his mind deteriorated, Ralph forgot that our children had grown up, married and moved away. On several occasions, he asked, "Where's Dennis?" He had forgotten that our son had passed away in 1967.

He often asked, "Where are the girls? Did they go somewhere?" He had also forgotten that the girls had gone away to college, married and moved out of state.

On June 15, 2000, Ralph fell off his chair while putting on his shoes. On June 17, he fell twice in the night when he got up to go to the bathroom.

I took him to see his family physician at Cambridge. He said to discontinue the Aricept medication and see his Neurologist at Zanesville.

The Neurologist started him on Exelon, the newest Alzheimer's medication.

Ralph's walking improved but the merciless disease continued to take its toll.

On Jun 19, he went to bed about 7 p.m. and at 9:30 he came downstairs dressed and said he was ready to go to the hay sale.

On July 10, he wanted to go home. I told him we were already home and took him out to the mailbox to show him our names on the mailbox.

On August 13, we attended a family reunion. Ralph sat down at the table and began to eat, ahead of everyone else. Soon after that, he wanted to go home. When he began walking toward the gate, I had to go after him and convince him that we would go home just as soon as I gathered up my things.

CHAPTER VII

WINTER IN WISCONSIN

By October, 2000, Ralph had begun to wander about the farm and walk along the road in front of our house. With winter coming on, I began to worry that he might get lost and it could be difficult to locate him after darkness set in. Also, the nights were growing cooler and if he were exposed to the cold night air for too long, hypothermia could develop. I did not wish to place him in a care center at that time, but found it difficult to keep track of him.

I discussed the situation with Janet and we decided that he might be better satisfied if we spent the winter with her in Wisconsin. She would be home all day and the two children also lived at home. She had a large house and there would be plenty of room for us. We decided it was the only alternative to placing him in a care center.

This time, we took a direct flight to the Minneapolis-St. Paul airport. Our grandson, Ben, met us there and drove us to River Falls where they live.

Things went quite well for a time, but Ralph gradually became agitated and confused. He wanted to go home and I tried to explain to him that our home was about one thousand miles away. However, he just shook his head and said, "No." He pointed to the hill back of their house. "It's just over that hill."

It was becoming more difficult for us to keep track of him there. He would walk outside and several times my granddaughter and I had to follow him and bring him back. On one occasion, he approached a neighbor who was outside in her yard and asked her to take him over town. I went to bring him back and explained to her that he had Alzheimer's.

Finally, my daughter and I came to the conclusion that it was not going to work out. We would either have to place him in a care center there, or, bring him back home to Ohio.

Ralph and I flew back to Columbus on November 14, 2000 and one of my nephews met us at the airport and drove us to our home near Newcomerstown.

HALLUCINATIONS?

At times, I thought he might be hallucinating. It became necessary to curtail our television viewing because he often thought the people on T.V. were actually here in our home, and, he was not going to bed as long as "those people" were here. Once, he became upset when we were watching a nature show and there were snakes on the T.V. I had to turn the T.V. off.

Once, he thought he had two cattle in the barn to sell. We hadn't had cattle for many years, and, I believe he saw two large round bales of hay inside the doorway and thought they were cattle.

On December 7, 2000, he became upset. When I asked him what was wrong, he replied, "We were on a boat and they took some people off; and, they took Mabel off and now I can't find her." He began to cry.

I believe his mind had flashed back to a deep-sea fishing trip we had taken in Florida.

CHAPTER VIII

A DIFFICULT DECISION

By the beginning of the year 2001, I began to think that Ralph had entered an advanced stage of the disease. He had been taking medications for Alzheimer's for more than five years, but, now he often didn't recognize me; he'd forgotten where he lived; he had stopped raising sweet corn; he had stopped hauling hay; and, he had stopped fishing, playing cards, and most of the other activities that he once enjoyed. He had recently begun to wander away from the house and, I feared that he might get lost and it would be difficult to locate him, especially in the evenings after darkness set in. I realized that I would be unable to care for him at home much longer.

Placing him in a care center was a difficult decision. But, Ralph seemed to understand that he needed more care than I could give him at home, alone. However, I did not wish to place him in a care center unless he was willing to go. I asked him if he wanted to live in a care center and, to my surprise, he said, "Yes."

I consulted his family physician and it was decided that Riverside Manor Rehabilitation and Care Center at Newcomerstown would be an ideal location. It was about three miles from our home and I could visit him every day.

Ralph was admitted to Riverside Manor on May 5, 2001. He adjusted quite well to his new surroundings. For the first few nights, his bed was moved out into the hallway where the nurse on duty could monitor him from the nurse's station.

I visited him every day and he seemed to be more satisfied there than he was at home. He enjoyed being around people and at home there had been few visitors. He enjoyed the movies they showed and the groups who came to entertain them. He was free to walk along the hallways, but the center did not have a secure unit for Alzheimer's patients and he walked outside a few times. However, the alarm on the door alerted the personnel and he was immediately returned.

After a few weeks, members of the family became concerned that, since he was always an avid fisherman, he might be attracted to the river which was nearby. Consequently, on May 25, we moved him to West Lafayette Rehabilitation and Nursing Center which has a locked-in unit for Alzheimer's patients.

CHAPTER IX

A NIGHTMARE

Soon after he was moved to West Lafayette, a series of events occurred which I can only describe as a "nightmare." I visited him daily and often had lunch there with him. He always seemed calm while I was with him, but the nurse said that he became agitated and pulled down curtains, shoved furniture and tried to get into other patients' rooms. I didn't observe any of this type of behavior while I was visiting him and I have concluded that it was a reaction to being suddenly confined in a locked-in unit. He had lived on a farm all of his life and had been free to move about anywhere and anytime he desired. I believe that being confined in a locked-in unit could have had a traumatic effect on him.

On June 2, the Care Center called and said they would like to send Ralph to Daybreak Center for Senior Psychiatric Services at Selby General Hospital, Marietta, Ohio for evaluation and treatment. They assured me that they had sent other patients there and when they returned they were calmer and easy to manage.

Of course my daughters and I wanted the best possible care for him, so we agreed. We trusted them to do what was best for him.

Although it was more than eighty miles from our home, I visited him several times. He was always calm, could walk about, feed himself and carry on a conversation while I was there. H e recognized his sister, her husband and me when we visited him.

THE AFFIDAVIT

On June 7, 2001, five days after he was admitted to Daybreak Center at Selby General Hospital, Marietta, I received a certified letter from the Washington County Court at Marietta. The letter contained a copy of an affidavit that had been filed in the court there. It alleged that my husband, Ralph, was mentally ill. A hearing had been scheduled for June 15, 2001, 8 a.m., and the court would decide if he were mentally ill and where he would be placed. Copies of this ten-page document were sent to: Ron Rees, Washington County Mental Health and Addiction Recovery Board; Michael G. Spahr, Washington County Prosecutor; Dr. Tony Byler, Affiant and CCO; Rolf Baumgartel, Attorney for Respondent; and Mabel Pollock, Spouse.

I was greatly troubled by this turn of events. Ralph's condition had been diagnosed in 1996 by a Florida Neurologist as Alzheimer's. I believe that Alzheimer's _IS_ a mental condition and many patients who have it become agitated and are usually treated with medications. I found it difficult to understand WHY they had scheduled a court hearing.

I immediately took the papers to the West Lafayette Rehabilitation and Nursing Center which had recommended sending him to Marietta and asked them what the papers meant.

The Administrator said that he had never seen the papers and knew nothing about them.

At that time, I became quite upset. I went home and called my daughter, Karen, in Florida. I told her about the papers and she placed a call to the Psychiatrist who had signed the forms. Her call was never returned. (Copies of these papers are included at the back of this book.)

On June 8, Ralph's sister and her husband accompanied me to Marietta. At the hospital, we questioned the nurse on duty about the papers. She said that they could cancel the hearing. However, she said that I should sign a voluntary admission form. At that point, I was not convinced that I should sign anything. My brother-in-law read the form and advised against it. Page 3 said that the patient may request in writing his release from the hospital. Then, the chief clinical officer of the hospital must either discharge him or file an affidavit for involuntary commitment within three court days of receipt of the letter requesting release. Of course Ralph was unable to write or sign his name, and I was not sure that he would be released if I signed the papers. Therefore, I declined to sign them at that time.

On our way home, Ralph's sister, her husband and I agreed that I needed legal advice. They recommended a lawyer friend of theirs and on June 13, I consulted him. He examined the papers and told me that, if the hearing were held, I would probably

44

lose control of Ralph's health care. Also, a lien could possibly be placed against our farm to pay for his care.

That night, I called my daughters and discussed the situation with them. We felt that we were quite capable of making decisions for his health care. We did not wish him placed in a mental institution far from his home. We loved him and wanted him placed where it would be convenient to visit him. Also, we expected to remain in control of his health care AND his assets.

Furthermore, we felt that it had not been necessary to schedule a court hearing. If it had become necessary to place him in a mental institution, we would have done so without a court order or hearing, and, we felt that we, alone, had the right to make that decision.

POWER OF ATTORNEY

Fortunately, in 1993, Ralph and I had made out Power of Attorney for Health Care papers to each other. If not for this, he might have been placed in an institution of the court's choosing without my consent and I might have lost control of his health care and, possibly, his assets.

With only two days remaining before the hearing, I had to act fast. I contacted Riverside Manor Rehabilitation and Care Center in Newcomerstown, where he had been placed originally, and explained the situation to them. I asked if they would take him back and they agreed. He had not given them any serious problems while he was a resident there before, and, his agitation could be controlled with proper medication.

I went to the bank and took my Power of Attorney for Health Care papers out of our Safe Deposit box. Then, I contacted my two brothers and they accompanied me to Daybreak Center at Selby General Hospital, Marietta. There, I showed my P.O.A. papers to the nurse on duty and told her that I had made arrangements to move Ralph to Riverside Manor at Newcomerstown. After she verified this, the hearing was cancelled and he was released.

CHAPTER X

BACK AT RIVERSIDE

During the ride back from Marietta in my car, Ralph was calm and never exhibited any signs of agitation. He rode in the front seat and one of my brothers drove. We arrived at the care center around 3:00 p.m. They had been expecting him. An aide came out with a wheelchair and wheeled him inside. She took him to his room and I stayed there with him until he became tired and went to sleep.

Ralph got along quite well at Riverside Manor. He seemed to remember being there before, and, he enjoyed being around other people, some of whom he formerly knew. He was free to walk about and he could still feed himself. He could still carry on a limited conversation and an alarm bracelet was placed around his wrist to alert the personnel when he attempted to go outside.

Ralph never complained, or begged me to take him home. I believe he had completely forgotten his home and thought the care center was his home.

I visited him every day and often had lunch with him there. He liked to walk about and, once, walked out onto the patio outside the dining area which has a fenced-in yard. While there, he stumbled on the cement and fell, bruising his temple.

On another occasion, he walked into the dining area where residents had been allowed to smoke earlier. He picked up an ashtray and began to eat the ashes. He was rushed to the hospital where it was determined that he had not eaten enough to harm him. I asked what would have happened if he had consumed a harmful amount and they said that he could have gone into convulsions.

After about three months, Riverside Manor informed me that Medicare would no longer pay for his care. The therapy was not doing him any good and he would be switched from skilled care to custodial care. This meant that we would have to pay for his care.

We had sold his machinery in June and we used this money to pay for his care. In addition to his room and board, I received bills which I considered huge from the Drug Company at New Philadelphia which supplied his medication.

I contacted the ombudsman and she conferred with the company and they agreed to cut the charges to the same amount they charge for Medicaid patients. In six months, I paid $4,536.33 for drugs, and, if I had not contested the charges, I would have had to pay $6,742.76.

When I learned that our four grandchildren were coming to visit "Grandpa" and attend the family reunion, I was elated. All three of the girls played piano and I began looking for a keyboard for them to play. I found a nice one at a garage sale and, after they arrived on August 11, 2001, we enjoyed it very much. We took it to the family reunion where they took turns playing it.

Soon after they arrived, we went to visit Ralph. I could see that he was pleased to see them. I believe he thought that Cheryl, our oldest granddaughter, was our daughter, Karen, because he called her "Karen." He called Sara, our youngest grandchild, "Janet," her mother's name. He called Christina, "Red." He had always liked to tease her about her red hair. He remembered Ben's name and was happy to see him.

Although the girls were visibly upset and cried over Ralph's emaciated appearance, I believe that he thoroughly enjoyed their visit and it lifted his spirits.

After the grandchildren went back to their homes, I began to play the keyboard. I had played the piano years ago when the children were young, but had not played much since then. However, I soon found that it was a great way to deal with some of the stress I have been under since Ralph became ill and I play it every day.

At Christmas time, the care center prepared a special dinner for the residents and their families. While we were dining, Ralph reached out and took a small, silver ornament from the centerpiece and attempted to put it into his mouth. I believe he thought it was candy.

On January 1, 2002, we celebrated his 81st birthday. The aides and I sang "Happy Birthday" to him. When one of them asked him how old he was, he replied, "I'm not so old."

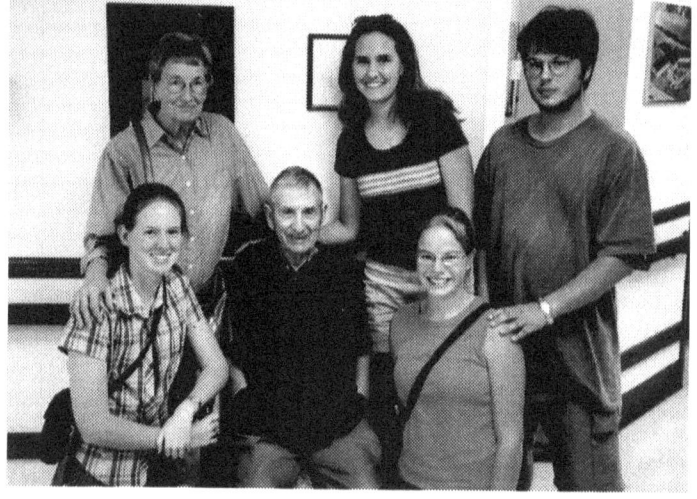

A visit from the grandchildren in August, 2001 lifted Ralph's spirits. Their visit also lifted my spirits and provided a welcome respite from the worry and anxiety associated with having a loved one who suffers from Alzheimer's disease.

PNEUMONIA & OTHER PROBLEMS

Ralph had been a resident of Riverside Manor for about eight months when, around the first of February, 2002, I noticed that his eyes didn't appear normal. He stared straight ahead and gave no indication that he saw me. He did not respond when I attempted to talk with him. The next day, he seemed the same and I thought that, perhaps I had visited at a time when he needed to sleep. However, on February 3, he still did not respond and I went to the Nurse's station and asked if he was alright. She checked his chart and said, "His vital signs are o.k."

The next morning, February 4, the Nurse called and said that Ralph had developed a temperature and high blood pressure. They wanted to send him to the hospital at Coshocton.

There, his condition was diagnosed as double pneumonia of the lower lobes; a stomach aneurysm of 4.5 centimeters; an infection of the urinary tract; high blood sugar; high blood pressure; dehydration; a temperature; plus, signs of a stroke which left him unable to swallow. He was hospitalized for eleven days and a gastrostomy tube for feeding was installed.

CHAPTER XI

AUTUMN HEALTH CARE

On February 15, Ralph was moved to Autumn Health Care at Coshocton, a skilled facility which was nearer to the hospital. This was advisable because of his condition.

He was placed in a semi-private room where he had a space of about six by six feet behind the door. I visited him every day and he usually recognized me. He was able to carry on a very limited conversation. He was given physical therapy and could walk a short distance with support on both sides; but, he remained in a wheelchair the balance of the time.

On May 16, 2002, I received a certified letter from Autumn Health Care which stated that Medicare would not cover his stay there as of May 5, and, he would be charged the private pay rate. According to the Medicare book, Medicare coverage ends the day after one receives the notice of non-coverage. Therefore I believed that Medicare ended May 16 instead of May 5. The letter also stated: Under a provision of the Medicare law, you do not have to pay for non-covered services determined to be custodial or not reasonable or necessary, unless you had reason to know the services were non-covered effective with the date of this notice.

BILLS, BILLS, BILLS

Soon after this, Autumn Health Care began to send me statements in which the charges went back to March 7, 2002. Instead of May 16, as their letter indicated. Included were charges of $2.72 for each 8-ounce can of Jevity, the liquid nutrition which Ralph needed. I could have purchased this product from a local distributor for much less and I was told by the distributor that, as long as Ralph couldn't swallow, Medicare would pay for it. After he was moved from Autumn Health Care, Medicare DID cover this charge. However, Autumn Health Care still included it in their bills, and, they made no adjustment for the cost of meals which he was unable to consume all of the time he was there, four months.

As of October 31, 2002, Autumn Care began to add interest at the rate of 1.5% compounded monthly onto the bill. As of July 31, 2003, the interest charges alone added up to $1,740.57.

Since I was concerned over the inaccuracy in the bills, I decided to contact the Department in Washington which oversees Medicare. On February 19, 2003, I received a reply from CMS AdminaStar Federal, a CMS Contracted Carrier and Intermediary. It was signed by Joe Carney, Analyst, Medicare Benefit Integrity

Unit. The letter stated that the matter would be investigated fully.

On March 19, 2003, I called CMS AdminaStar and learned that they had not started the investigation as of that time. On May 5, I called again and talked with Kevin Bartow who said it would be late June or early July before they could get to it. I told him that they were charging interest at the rate of 1½ percent, compounded each month (18% per year) and he said that they could not charge interest as long as the account is under investigation.

I called again around the first of July and Bartow said it would be October before they could get around to it because they had more than 2,500 other cases to investigate.

Early in December, I received a call from a representative of CMS AdminaStar informing me that the investigation would take place before long and I would be notified of the results. As of January 5, 2004, I have received no further correspondence. Copies of Autumn Health Care's letter, a list of their bills, and a copy of the letter from CMS, AdminaStar Federal are included at the back of this book. In February, this issue was resolved and the account paid in full.

CHAPTER XII

HOME AGAIN

Due to the controversy over the bills and the high cost of keeping him in a small 6 x 6 foot space behind a door, I decided to care for Ralph at home. He was now in a wheelchair full time and he couldn't wander away from the house as he did before. Also, I suspected that he was in an advanced stage of the disease and I felt that it would be more satisfactory for both of us if he could spend the balance of his days at home.

I had a ramp installed at the front door so that we could wheel him outside for fresh air every day. I rented a hospital bed from a local medical equipment dealer. I learned to feed him his Jevity through his stomach tube. And, I located two women who were willing to help care for him part time.

On June 17, 2002, we brought Ralph home. The Coshocton Health Care Agency was very helpful. They sent a nurse to check his condition at least once a week; a therapist who came twice a week and soon had him standing and walking a short distance with support. And, an aide came twice a week to bathe him. I gave him his Jevity six times a day and Medicare covered the cost of everything including his Jevity.

In the beginning, I thought the arrangement was working out quite well; but, before long, I realized that Ralph had advanced to a stage where he was uncooperative. When I tried to move him from the wheelchair to the bed; or, from the bed to the wheelchair, he would resist and occasionally kicked at me. Sometimes he would also make a fist.

When I was alone with him and tried to roll him over while getting him ready for bed, he would grasp the bed-rail and hold on with a grip that I had difficulty loosening.

At times, he would scoot about the house in his wheelchair and, several times he slid out of it onto the floor. Then, it was impossible for me to get him up and I had to call someone to help me.

By the end of three weeks, I was becoming exhausted, both physically and mentally. I did not want to admit that I was unable to care for him properly at home; but I knew that to continue that regimen for long would eventually affect my own health.

At such a late stage, Ralph had completely forgotten that this was his home, and that I was his wife. He had become accustomed to being around other people, and he had few visitors here. I decided that he would be better satisfied in a care center.

CHAPTER XIII

BELL NURSING HOME

I contacted Bell Nursing Home at Kimbolton and they sent a caseworker to make an assessment of Ralph's needs. She recommended a care center and arrangements were made to place him in Bell Nursing Home. It was my first choice because one of my brothers lives near there and I knew that he would visit Ralph often. That would be of great help and comfort to me.

It was decided that he should have a check-up before being moved and, on the afternoon of July 8, 2002, two of my brothers helped me take him to his local doctor. His condition was described as "severe" Alzheimer's and we moved him directly from the doctor's office to the care center.

Ralph got along better than I expected in his new "home." The staff was very caring and some of the aides began to call him

"Grandpa." I visited him every day, except when I had a cold. Other visitors included my three brothers, my sister, nephew, and, his brother. Bob. However, I don't believe he recognized any of them except my younger brother. Ralph smiled when Homer talked to him about the many fishing trips they had taken together.

One day as we sat in the lobby of the care center, I noticed that Ralph was admiring the beautiful, marble fireplace there. "Is this your home?" I asked and he replied, "Yes." I knew then that it would be his final home.

Ralph seemed to enjoy sitting in the lobby and watching Country & Western shows on television. A few times, I took my keyboard and played some toe-tapping music for him and some of the other residents there. They seemed to enjoy it.

In an effort to jog his memory, I often took family pictures to show him, but he failed to identify most of them. However, when I showed him a snapshot of the two of us taken several years earlier in Florida, I asked him, "Do you know the woman in this picture?"

He looked at it a moment then replied, "That's my wife, Mabel."

"Good," I said. I was elated. "And," I continued, "who is that man with her?"

He studied the picture for a moment, then replied, "That's what I'd like to know."

A VISIT FROM KAREN

In October, 2002, Karen and I made plans to travel to Wisconsin to visit Janet, who has had multiple sclerosis for more than four years and is in a care center there. Neither of us had seen her in more than two years and we considered it a trip of necessity. Furthermore, we wanted to make our trip before the cold weather began.

Of course, I was concerned about leaving Ralph; but he was in good hands and we would be gone for only a few days. We left our cell phone number with the Nursing home and planned to check on him every day. If there were an emergency, we would return immediately.

I met Karen at the Columbus airport and, from there we drove directly to Wisconsin. We had a wonderful visit with Janet, her son and daughter. I had been concerned that Janet might be depressed over her father's condition; but, I believe our visit lifted her spirits and it was good therapy for all of us.

Karen and I returned from Wisconsin on Saturday evening, October 26, 2002. We drove directly to Bell Nursing Home to see Ralph. We found him sitting in his wheelchair, just inside his room.

"Hello, Ralph," I said as we entered. "There is someone with me who wants to see you."

His eyes widened in surprise as he saw Karen for the first time since our last trip to Florida in 1999. I was glad to see that he recognized her.

Karen went over to him and gave him a big hug. As I watched, I could see a tear build up in the corner of his eye and slide down his cheek. Even though he was in an advanced stage of the disease, he was still capable of emotional feelings.

The next morning, about 3:30 a.m., Karen and I were awakened by the sound of stones hitting the house and the breaking of glass.

We hurried to the window, but the vehicle sped away before we could get a description. We called the Sheriff's office and an examination of the house revealed that stones had been thrown with enough force to break the window glass, scattering glass onto the bed which, fortunately, was unoccupied. The perpetrators of this Halloween prank were never caught, but, needless to say, we were quite upset over this uncivilized act and were unable to sleep for several nights.

The next day, October 27, the Nursing Home called and said that Ralph was not feeling well and they wanted to send him to Southeastern Ohio Regional Medical Center at Cambridge. Karen and I drove to the hospital right away. Ralph was still in the emergency room and we had to wait to see him. Finally, the doctor came out and told us that he had pneumonia. (Aspirational pneumonia seems to be a common side effect of tube feeding.)

He was started on antibiotics and hospitalized for two weeks. After he recovered, he was returned to Bell Nursing Home. Later, an X-ray revealed that he also had COPD (chronic obstructive pulmonary disease.)

After Karen returned to Miami, Ralph didn't seem to remember that she had been to visit him. I believe he had entered a very advanced stage of the disease.

By the end of 2002, Ralph was no longer able to sit in a wheelchair. He was placed in a Geri-chair which was moved about, usually into the lobby where he seemed to enjoy watching Country and Western shows on television, or, into the dining area when there were entertainers visiting.

"LITTLE BIRD"

As winter approached, the house seemed strangely quiet. At times I felt as if I were stranded on an island in the middle of nowhere. I literally threw myself into my writing, and, when I felt stressed, I played the keyboard. I visited Ralph every day and often had lunch with him. I joined the Senior Center at Newcomerstown and went there often for companionship.

At night, it had become my custom to close the drapes as darkness set in. One night in late November, as I pulled the shade over the kitchen window, I noticed a small shape huddled in the corner of the awning. I took a second look and recognized it as a sparrow. The next morning, I raised the shade and the bird flew away.

Every night, before I went to bed, I checked the awning and noticed that the sparrow had returned and every morning it would fly away. I began to call it "Little Bird" and looked forward to its company. It reminded me of the song, "His Eye Is On The Sparrow," and I know He watches me.

Often a second sparrow would perch in the opposite corner of the awning. I believe they were a pair. All winter long one or both of the sparrows would spend the night on the narrow ledge of the awning. When the weather became stormy, the birds did not appear. They probably spent those nights in an outbuilding nearby.

One morning in early spring, "Little Bird" flew away and that night she didn't return. I checked the awning every night and, when she still did not appear, I decided that she and her mate had flown to a tree, or perhaps the barn to build a nest and raise a family.

About two months later, "Little Bird" reappeared in the corner of the awning. This time, she stayed for about two months, then flew away again. I wondered if she had flown to the hill to find another tree to build another nest and raise a second family before the cold weather began.

Each night, I checked the awning and thought that, this time, she had left permanently; but, on September 12, 2003, as I pulled the shade over the window, I noticed a familiar, gray shape in the corner of the awning. My spirits lifted. "Little Bird" had returned and, this time, I believe she will spend the winter with me.

CHAPTER XIV

HIS FINAL DAYS

Around the first of February, 2003, Ralph developed pneumonia for the third time within a year. It was decided to keep him in the Nursing home instead of sending him to the hospital. He was given antibiotics through his feeding tube.

Each day I visited him, but the antibiotics did not seem to be taking effect as they had before. He grew more lethargic each day and did not respond when I attempted to talk with him. As his breathing grew more and more laborious, I became alarmed and called our daughters to inform them that he was not doing well. They were concerned about my welfare and urged me to get as much rest as possible.

On February 7th, I sat with him all afternoon. He held so tightly onto my hand that it hurt. It seemed as if he didn't want to let go. Finally, he drifted into a fitful sleep. At that time, I began to think that I might be called in the middle of the night, so I decided that it would be best if I went home and got some rest. The nurse in charge said that she would call me if there were any change in his condition.

The call came sooner than I had expected. I arrived at the Nursing home about 10:00 p.m., but Ralph had passed away about ten minutes earlier. I felt remorseful over not being with him at the end. Had I known the call would come so soon, I would have remained there with him.

The aide who attended him said that he went peacefully. She was very caring and treated him like a member of her own family. She called him "Grandpa."

Ralph's funeral was held February 11, 2003. That was the day we would have celebrated our 60th wedding anniversary, if a cure for his disease had been developed in time.

Our daughter, Janet, who has had multiple sclerosis for more than four years, was unable to attend the funeral, but, her son and daughter came. Janet faxed the eulogy which was read by Karen who added some thoughts of her own as well as those of her two daughters.

Ralph is at peace now. There is no more confusion, no more forgetfulness, and, no more agitation. He lived a good life until he reached the late stage of Alzheimer's. I am thankful that he had 82 years, and that most of those years, except for the last two, were good quality, productive years.

During the late stage of the disease, it was often upsetting when he couldn't remember me. We had lived together for almost sixty years and the disease had wiped out most of his memory of that time. However, I take comfort in knowing that, the next time we meet, he will recognize me instantly.

MY OWN CONCLUSIONS

In conclusion, I would like to add that I believe that more should be done to pinpoint the causes of many diseases and to develop cures for them. Victims of these diseases do not have years to wait for cures. They need them now.

A few years ago, exciting results from embryonic stem-cell research brought new hope to many victims of diseases. According to reports on auto-immune diseases and stem-cell based therapies, there is evidence that embryonic stem-cells are preferable to adult stem-cells because they can develop into all organs of the body; they are more receptive to genetic manipulation than adult stem-cells; and, preliminary findings raise the possibility that lines derived from embryonic stem-cells may be less susceptible to rejection by the recipient's immune system than lines derived from adult stem-cells.

Where will these embryonic stem-cells come from? According to reports, there are approximately 400,000 frozen embryos stored in fertility clinics' freezers. These were created to enable women who were unable to conceive, to bear children. Extra embryos were created to insure success. Usually, only one embryo is implanted inside a woman's womb and the extra embryos must eventually be destroyed. The extra embryos should be made available to laboratories for stem-cell research.

There is basically no difference between using stem-cells from an extra embryo which is scheduled to be destroyed than using organs from the bodies of persons who have been fatally injured in accidents. It is possible that some of the opponents of embryonic stem-cell use may be recipients of organ transplants. Why should we place a higher value on an embryo which is scheduled to be destroyed than on the life of a person who has a disease for which stem-cells from that same embryo might provide a cure?

I believe that, if embryonic stem-cell research had been approved and funded by our government at the time the first stem-cell was isolated, cures for many diseases may have been developed by now. Meanwhile, thousands of victims of Alzheimer's, Parkinson's, multiple sclerosis, cancer, diabetes and other ailments continue to suffer and die prematurely.

Although embryonic stem-cell research has been greatly curtailed in the United States, it continues unabated in private laboratories which do not receive Federal funds, and in countries such as Canada, England, Sweden, Israel, China and others. Hopefully, scientists in these countries and in private laboratories will soon develop cures for many diseases and share these cures with the rest of the world.

In addition to medical research, I believe that more studies should be made to determine whether some conditions are genetic, or are possibly caused by environmental factors.

WATER: When America was first settled, our rivers and streams were clear and pure enough to use for drinking and cooking. Today, it is considered unsafe to eat the fish from some of these waterways due to contamination. Many of our water sources and private wells have become contaminated and, today, bottled water has become a growing industry.

AIR: The ozone layer which shields us from the ultraviolet rays which are known to cause skin cancer, is being gradually depleted by exhausts from automobiles, aerosol products and other sources.

MEDICATIONS: Unproven medications can lead to disastrous results. Several years ago, thalidomide, a prescription drug used by pregnant women to prevent morning sickness, resulted in babies born with physical abnormalities.

CHEMICALS: Several years ago, members of families who built their homes on a reclaimed dump site at the Love Canal in New York where toxic chemicals had been disposed of, became ill and were forced to move.

Agent Orange, the chemical used by the U.S. Army to defoliate forests during the Vietnam conflict, has been blamed by many veterans who were exposed to it for their health problems.

Chemical sprays used on lawns, gardens and farm fields are toxic and, if not used properly, can lead to health problems.

The United States is reported to have a huge supply of nerve gas in its arsenal. To my knowledge, there has not been developed a safe method to dispose of it.

RADIATION: There have been nuclear accidents. The worst of these was the Chernobyl accident in Russia which rendered a huge area unsafe for human habitation for many years to come.

Recently, it was reported that some Nevada residents are vigorously opposed to a plan to transport radioactive wastes cross-country to a cave near their town where it will be sealed and buried. It was reported that these wastes may remain radioactive for as long as 25,000 years. 25,000 years? And, more will accumulate every day.

In retrospect, it seems a bit short-sighted on the part of all world leaders to allow any dangerous product to be manufactured and placed on the market before an antidote, or control is developed for it. If a method cannot be developed to neutralize it, then, its use should be banned.

Will we leave a safe and healthy world for future generations; or, will greed and selfishness lead to our downfall?

SUGGESTIONS FOR THE CAREGIVER

1. Always keep in mind that Alzheimer's is caused by cells dying in the brain at a faster than normal rate. The mind gradually regresses back to childhood, or earlier.

2. Don't scold him or her when he does things that irritate you. Always remember that "he can't help it."

3. Don't discuss his condition with others in his presence. He may be able to understand more than you realize.

4. Find an outlet for the stress caused by caring for a person who is agitated or mentally confused. If possible, at least once a week take him to a day care center, then visit a friend, go shopping, or find a hobby which you will enjoy. I began to play the keyboard and joined the local Senior Center where I can socialize with other people. I also write books, and, this is my third one.

5.   Don't jeopardize your own health trying to "do your duty." Gone are the days when families were large and there was plenty of help available when needed. Today, it is usually the spouse alone who must shoulder the full responsibility, not only of caring for the patient, but of maintaining the home, seeing that the grass is mowed, taking care of all paperwork connected with his health care, finding the means to pay taxes, car upkeep, car insurance, health insurance, home insurance, and other bills on an income that was practically depleted when he became ill.

6.   Protect the patient's legal rights. Make sure your loved one has made out a Power of Attorney to a reliable, honest family member, or to someone who can be completely trusted. Alzheimer's victims often become targets for unscrupulous individuals who prey upon the elderly, especially when assets are involved. Be extra cautious before signing any papers. If there is even an iota of doubt in your mind, get a second, or third opinion before signing anything.

7. Maintain a sense of humor if you can. I laughed when my husband came downstairs wearing my white slacks and blouse. I laughed when he said he was going to marry me. I laughed when I showed him a picture of the two of us and asked him who the man was with me, and he replied, "That's what I'd like to know."

8. Finally, when the patient no longer recognizes you, doesn't remember where he lives, and needs 24-hour a day care, if you are still trying to care for him at home, it is time to consider placing him in a facility where he will be well cared for. He will probably be happier there than he was at home, and it will give you greater peace of mind. Then, perhaps your blood pressure will return to normal again, as mine did.

Mabel V. Pollock

APPENDIX

The following copies of the affidavit from Probate Court, Washington County, Ohio, and copies of bills from Autumn Health Care, Coshocton, Ohio, as well as copies of correspondence with Health Care Financing Administration, Washington, D.C., are included to illustrate just how complicated the paperwork for Medicare and Care Centers can be for 70, 80 or even 90 year old patients, or their spouses, who are expected to, somehow, cope with these problems and find the means to pay these bills.

Mabel V. Pollock

IN THE COURT OF COMMON PLEAS
PROBATE COURT
WASHINGTON COUNTY, OHIO

In the Matter of:	)	Case No.: 2001 MN 00014
	)	
RALPH POLLOCK	)	NOTICE OF HEARING
Alleged to be Mentally Ill	)	

FILED
JUN - 6 2001
TIMOTHY A. WILLIAMS, JUDGE
PROBATE COURT
WASHINGTON COUNTY, OHIO

TO THE FOLLOWING PERSONS:

1. Ron Rees, Washington County Mental   regular mail to 109 Scammel St., Marietta, OH
   Health & Addiction Recovery Board

2. Michael G. Spahr,   hand delivered by Deputy Clerk
   Washington County Prosecutor

3. Dr. Tony Byler, Affiant & COO   hand delivered by Sheriff's Office

4. Rolf Baumgartel,   placed in court box
   Attorney for Respondent

5. Mabel Pollock, spouse   regular mail to: 21291 Twp. Rd. 257,
                                         Newcomerstown, OH 43832

This matter is set for hearing before this Court at Daybreak Center

For Senior Psychiatric Services, Selby General Hospital, 1106 Colegate

Drive, Marietta, OH

on the 15th day of _____June_____ , 20 01 , at 8:00

o'clock a .m.

Witness my signature and the seal
of said Court, this 6th day
of ____June____ ＊ , 20 01

(seal)

TIMOTHY A. WILLIAMS

Probate Judge/Magistrate

Trish Whitley
Deputy Clerk

TO: Respondent's Legal Guardian/Adult Next of Kin
    Respondent's Spouse
    Respondent's parents, (minor child)
    Affiant
    Respondent's Counsel
    Chief Clinical Officer
    Community Mental Health Board

IN THE COURT OF COMMON PLEAS
PROBATE COURT
WASHINGTON COUNTY, OHIO

AFFIDAVIT (MENTAL ILLNESS)

Pollock, Ralph

FILED

Case Number
2001 MN 00014

JUN 6 2001

TIMOTHY A. WILLIAMS, JUDGE
PROBATE COURT
WASHINGTON COUNTY, OHIO

The State of Ohio, Washington County, S.S.

Tony Byler, MD, ~~DAVID HILL, MD~~ the undersigned, residing at *701 Hildreth Lane, Marietta, OH*, says that he has information to believe, or has actual knowledge that *Ralph Pollock*, a resident of Coschoton County is mentally ill and ....

Represents a substantial risk of physical harm to himself as manifested by evidence of threats of, or attempts at, suicide or serious self-inflicted bodily harm;

✓ Represents a substantial risk of physical harm to others as manifested by evidence of recent homicidal or other violent behavior or evidence of recent threats that place another in reasonable fear of violent behavior and serious physical harm;

Represents a substantial and immediate risk of physical impairment or injury to herself/himself as manifested by evidence that he is unable to provide for and is not providing for her/his basic physical needs because of mental illness and that appropriate provision for such needs cannot be made immediately available in The community; or

Would benefit from treatment in a hospital for his mental illness and is in need of such treatment in a hospital for his mental illness and is in need of such treatment as manifested by evidence of behavior that creates a grave and imminent risk to substantial rights of others or himself.
(Specify specific category or categories above with X)   *

Tony Byler, MD/ ~~DAVID HILL, MD~~ further says that the facts supporting this belief are as follows:

Patient is demented and very violent to peers and staff.

These facts being sufficient to indicate probable cause that the above said person is a mentally ill person subject to hospitalization by Court order.

R.C. 5122.15

IN THE MATTER OF

RALPH POLLOCK

CASE NO: 2001 MN 00014

ALLEGED TO BE MENTALLY ILL

(B)   Unless the Court finds by clear and convincing evidence that the respondent is M.I., and subject to hospitalization by Court Order, it shall order immediate discharge, unless conditional release is ordered pursuant to Section 2945.40(D).

(C)   If the Court finds that the respondent is M.I. and subject to hospitalization, the Court shall order the respondent for a period not to exceed 90 days, to one of the following:

  (1)   a hospital operated by the D.M.H. if the respondent is committed pursuant to section 2945.38 (D), or Section 2945.40, 5120.17, or 5139.08 of the O.R.C.

  (2)   a nonpublic hospital.

  (3)   The V.A. or other agency of the U.S. Government.

  (4)   A C.M.H.B., or an agency that the Board designates.

  (5)   To receive private psychiatric or psychological care and treatment.

  (6)   Any other suitable facility, or person consistent with the needs of the respondent.

That the name and address of respondent's legal guardian, spouse and adult next of kin are:

Name	Kinship	Address
	Legal Guardian	
Mabel Pollock	Spouse	21291 Township 257 Newcomerstown, OH 740-498-7390

That the following constitutes additional information that may be necessary for the purpose of

determining residence.   N/A

Dated this **6 th**   day of **June**   A.D., 2001

Affiant

Tony Byler, MD/ ~~David Hill, MD~~

Sworn to before me and signed in my presence on the day and year above dated

Pro̶b̶a̶t̶e̶ J̶u̶d̶g̶e̶/Notary Public

Deputy Clerk

Waiver

I, the undersigned affiant, hereby waive the issuing and service of Notice of the Hearing on said
Affidavit, and voluntarily enter my appearance herein.

Dated   2001

Affiant

IN THE COURT OF COMMON PLEAS
PROBATE DIVISION
WASHINGTON COUNTY, OHIO

IN THE MATTER OF)
)
RALPH POLLOCK)   Case No.: 2001 MN 00014
ALLEGED TO BE MENTALLY ILL)

ORDER OF DETENTION

FILED

JUN - 6 2001

TIMOTHY A. WILLIAMS, JUDGE
PROBATE COURT
WASHINGTON COUNTY, OHIO

To: Robert R. Schlicher, Sheriff of said County:

Whereas, Dr. Tony Byler

who ~~resides~~at/works at Daybreak Center For Senior Psychiatric

Services, Selby General Hospital, 1106 Colegate Drive, Marietta, OH,

has filed an affidavit alleging that Ralph Pollock

~~residingxat~~/an inpatient at Daybreak Center For Senior Psychiatric

Services, Selby General Hospital, 1106 Colegate Drive, Marietta, OH,

is a mentally ill person subject to hospitalization by Court order.

Pursuant to Section 5122.11 of the Revised Code, the Court finds

probable cause to believe that respondent is a mentally ill person

subject to hospitalization by court order.

    You are, therefore, commanded to apprehend the said person

forthwith and detain him at Daybreak Center For Senior Psychiatric

Services, Selby General Hospital, 1106 Colegate Drive, Marietta, OH,

then and there to abide the order of this Court in the premises.

Herein fail not, and of this writ make legal services and due

return not later than the first business day after service is had.

In testimony thereof, I hereunto set
my hand and affix the seal of said
Probate Court at Marietta, Ohio.
This 6th   day of ___June___
A.D. 20 01

(seal)

Timothy A. Williams, Probate Judge

Deputy Clerk

-MN4-

IN THE COURT OF COMMON PLEAS
PROBATE COURT
WASHINGTON COUNTY, OHIO

In the Matter of

RALPH POLLOCK
Alleged to be Mentally Ill

)
)
)
)

Case No.: 2001 MN 00014

FILED

JUN - 6 2001

TIMOTHY A. WILLIAMS, JUDGE
PROBATE COURT
WASHINGTON COUNTY, OHIO

NOTICE TO RESPONDENT

Ralph Pollock
c/o Daybreak Center For Sr. Psych. Services
Selby General Hospital
1106 Colegate Drive
Marietta, OH 45750

You are hereby notified that on the 6th day of June ,
2001 , Dr. Tony Byler , xxxxdxxxxxxxx/who works at

Daybreak Center For Senior Psychiatric Services, Selby General Hospital,
1106 Colegate Drive, Marietta, OH 45750

filed in this Court an affidavit/xxxxxxxxxxxxxxxxxxxxxxxxxxxx
xxxxxxxxxxx alleging that you are mentally ill. This affidavit/
xxxxxxxxxxx will be for hearing before this Court at Daybreak Center For
Senior Psychiatric Services, Selby General Hospital, 1106 Colegate Dr., Marietta, OH,

on the 15th day of June , 2001 , at 8:00 a.m.

You may retain counsel and have independent expert evaluation.
If you are unable to obtain an attorney, you shall be represented
by court appointed counsel and may have independent expert
evaluation at state expense. You may select any one person upon
whom written notice of this hearing shall be served. Attorney

Rolf Baumgartel, WesBanco Bldg., Suite 206, 200 Putnam   Phone: (740)373-2420
Street, Marietta, OH 45750
has been appointed to represent you at this hearing.

Witness my signature and the seal
of said Court on this 6th day of
June , 20 01

(seal)

Timothy A. Williams
Probate Judge

Trish Whiteley
Deputy Clerk

-- MN7 --

IN THE COURT OF COMMON PLEAS
PROBATE DIVISION

IN THE MATTER OF	)	
	)	
RALPH POLLOCK	)	Case No.: 2001 MN 00014
	)	
ALLEGED TO BE MENTALLY ILL	)	

RIGHTS OF AN INVOLUNTARILY DETAINED PERSON

1. You have been taken into custody by _____
    _____ a ___Deputy Sheriff_____
    of Washington County, Ohio for transportation to an agency
    for examination by mental health professionals at the
    Daybreak Center For Senior Psychiatric Services, Selby General Hospital .
    This is not a criminal arrest.

2. You have the RIGHT to:

    a) MAKE immediately a REASONABLE NUMBER of TELEPHONE CALLS
        or use other reasonable means to contact an attorney,
        a physician, a licensed clinical psychologist, or to
        contact some other person or persons to secure represent-
        ation by counsel, or to obtain medical or psychological
        assistance, and be provided assistance in making calls
        if such assistance is needed and requested;

    b) RETAIN COUNSEL and have independent expert evaluation
        of your mental condition and, if you are unable to
        afford an attorney, be represented by Court-Appointed
        Counsel and have independent expert evaluation of your
        mental condition at public expense if you are unable
        to afford that evaluation;

    c) HAVE A HEARING to determine whether or not you are a
        mentally ill person subject to hospitalization by Court
        order;

    d) REQUEST A VOLUNTARY ADMISSION to this hospital which
        if accepted will result in an expungment of your Court
        record, if you voluntarily admit yourself before or at
        your initial hearing. Your Court file will also be
        expunged if at your initial hearing you are found not
        to be mentally ill subject to hospitalization by Court
        order.

REPORT OF PRESENTATION OF RIGHTS

On the _6th_ day of _____June_____ , 20_01_ , I read and
served a copy of RIGHTS OF AN INVOLUNTARILY DETAINED PERSON to
Ralph Pollock, an inpatient at Daybreak Center For Senior Psychiatric Services,
Selby General Hospital, 1106 Colegate Drive, Marietta, OH 45750.

_____
~~SHERIFF~~/DEPUTY SHERIFF/~~BAILIFF~~

-MN8-

IN THE COURT OF COMMON PLEAS
PROBATE DIVISION
WASHINGTON COUNTY, OHIO

IN THE MATTER OF: :

RALPH POLLOCK   : CASE NO. 2001 MN 00014

                     :

ALLEGED TO BE MENTALLY ILL   :

JOURNAL ENTRY SETTING HEARING ON AFFIDAVIT

The Court sets _____ June 13, 10 _____, 2001, at 8:00 o'clock a. m., as the

date and time for hearing the above captioned case. Said hearing to be conducted at the

DAYBREAK CENTER FOR SENIOR PSYCHIATRIC SERVICES, SELBY GENERAL

HOSPITAL, 1106 COLEGATE DRIVE, MARIETTA, OHIO, 45750.

ENTER AS OF THE DATE OF FILING

HON. TIMOTHY A. WILLIAMS
Probate Judge/Magistrate

-MNJ3SGH-

IN THE COURT OF COMMON PLEAS
PROBATE DIVISION
WASHINGTON COUNTY, OHIO

In The Matter of   )

)

RALPH POLLOCK   )   Case No.: 2001 MN 00014

)

Alleged to be Mentally Ill   )

                            JUDGMENT ENTRY
                            CONTINUANCE

    This matter came on for hearing pursuant to Sections

5122.141/5122.15 (H) of the Ohio Revised Code this   6th   day

of   June, 2001   ,   .

    For good cause shown, the hearing is ORDERED continued until

        June 15, 2001, at 8:00 a.m.   .

June 6, 2001
Date   Probate Judge/~~Magistrate~~
                            HON. TIMOTHY A. WILLIAMS

- MNI14 -

IN THE COURT OF COMMON PLEAS

PROBATE COURT

WASHINGTON COUNTY, OHIO

IN THE MATTER OF:)

RALPH POLLOCK   )   Case No.: 2001 MN 00014

ALLEGED TO BE MENTALLY ILL   )

JOURNAL ENTRY APPOINTING COUNSEL

As provided for in Section 5122.15 (A) of the Revised
Code and it further appearing to the Court that respondent
is unable to obtain counsel or is indigent, the Court
hereby orders that _____Rolf Baumgartel_____,
Attorney at Law, Marietta, Ohio, is appointed to act as
counsel in this matter. In the event that the above
captioned person is not indigent, the Court reserves the
right to assess costs to said person.

HON. TIMOTHY A. WILLIAMS
Probate Judge

-MN15-

Name & Location of Facility Selby Daybreak Behavioral Health Unit 1106 Colegate, Marietta, OH 45750	Date of Application June 13, 2001	
Name of Applicant Ralph L. Pollock	Social Security Number	Date of Birth 1-1-1921
Address (street, city, state, zip code) 21291 T.R. 257 Newcomerstown, Ohio 43832		
Applicant's County of Residence Coshocton		

Application

To the Chief Clinical Officer:

In accordance with the provisions of the Revised Code of Ohio, application is hereby made for such care and treatment that may be necessary in promoting the recovery of the patient.

It is specifically understood and agreed that if the patient is admitted to the hospital as a voluntary patient:

1.   That the patient will abide by all rules and regulations of the hospital.

2.   That the patient will leave the hospital on the request of the Chief Clinical Officer of the hospital, if the patient requires different care of treatment than that provided by the hospital.

3.   That the patient may request in writing his/her release from the hospital. The Chief Clinical Officer of the hospital then must either discharge the patient forthwith or file an affidavit for involuntary commitment within three court days of receipt of the letter requesting release.

Signature of Patient
Signature of Guardian or POA x *Mabel V. Pollock P.O.A.*

Signed in the presence of:

Witness *Jo Edwards, RN*	Witness *Linda Sintrunk MS, LSW*

Note: If patient is an adult incompetent, the application must be signed by his/her guardian or by the person having POA.

Approved ___ Yes ___ No	Signature of Chief Clinical Officer	Date

IN THE COURT OF COMMON PLEAS
PROBATE DIVISION
WASHINGTON COUNTY, OHIO

IN THE MATTER OF:)
)
RALPH POLLOCK   )
)   CASE NO.:   2001 MN 00014
ALLEGED TO BE MENTALLY ILL   )
)

FILED

JUN 1 4 2001

TIMOTHY A. WILLIAMS, JUDGE
PROBATE COURT
WASHINGTON COUNTY, OHIO

JUDGMENT ENTRY - ORDER OF DISMISSAL

The Court finds that this matter should be dismissed for the following reason:

XXX   The conditions justifying involuntary commitment no longer exist and the
             Respondent was discharged on _____June 14, 2001_____
             pursuant to Section 5122.21 of the Revised Code.

_____   The statutory time requirement for a mandatory full hearing pursuant to Section
              5122.15 of the Revised Code has not been met.

_____   The Respondent / Respondent's Medical Power of Attorney signed a Voluntary
              Admission.

        THEREFORE IT IS ORDERED that this cause should be and is hereby dismissed.

June 14, 2001
Date   TIMOTHY A. WILLIAMS, PROBATE JUDGE

-MN17A-

Copy to:
Ron Rees, WCMHARB
Michael G. Spahr
Rolf Baumgartel
√ Mabel Pollock

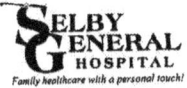

SELBY GENERAL HOSPITAL

Family healthcare with a personal touch!

June 14, 2001

Honorable Timothy A. Williams
Probate Court
Marietta Court House
Marietta, OH 45750

Honorable Williams:

RE: Ralph Pollock
        Cancel Probate Court Hearing
        Discharge Date: June 14, 2001

This is to notify you that Ralph Pollock was discharged from our unit this date at 1000 hours. It is no longer necessary to complete the involuntary admission process. Please cancel the hearing for Mr. Pollock that was scheduled for 15th at 8:00 a.m.

Sincerely,

Jenanne Leary-Rodriguez, RN
Program Administrator

www.selbygeneralhospital.com
1106 Colegate Drive, Marietta, OH 45750
740/568-2000
A teaching hospital accredited by the American Osteopathic Association.

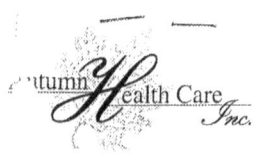

5/3/02

Mabel Pollock
21291 TR 257
Newcomerstown, OH 43832

Dear Mabel,

On 5/3/02 our Utilization Review Committee reviewed medical information and found that the services furnished for Ralph no longer qualifies for payment by Medicare beginning 5/5/02. The reason for this is: Medicare covers medically necessary skilled care needed on a daily basis. Skilled nursing care was needed beginning 2/15/02 to observe and evaluate his condition. Since skilled nursing care or skilled rehabilitation services are no longer needed on a daily basis, we believe his stay after 5/4/02 is not covered under Medicare.

This decision has not been made by Medicare. It represents the Utilization Review Committee's judgment that the services needed have no longer met Medicare payment requirements. A bill will be sent to Medicare for the covered services received before 5/5/02.
Normally, the bill submitted to Medicare does not include services provided after this date. If you want to appeal this decision, a request that the bill be submitted to Medicare includes the services our URC determined to be uncovered. Medicare will notify you of its determination. If you disagree with that determination, you may file an appeal.

Under a provision of the Medicare Law, you do not have to pay for non-covered services determined to be custodial or not reasonable or necessary, unless you had reason to know the services were non-covered effective with the date of this notice.

Please check one of the lines on the enclosed Request For Medicare Intermediary Review to indicate whether or not the bill for services after 5/4/02 be submitted to Medicare and sign the notice to verify receipt. Please return in the self-addressed stamped envelope at your earliest convenience. Thank you for your attention in this matter.

Sincerely yours,

Amy Dotson

Amy Dotson
Accounting Assistant

Autumn Health Care Inc.

3201 County Road 10
Coshocton, Ohio 43812

14
5-16-02

RETURN RECEIPT
REQUESTED

Mabel Pollock
31291 TR 257
Newcomerstown, OH
43832

CERTIFIED MAIL

PLACE STICKER AT TOP OF ENVELOPE
TO THE RIGHT OF RETURN ADDRESS,
FOLD AT DOTTED LINE

UNITED STATES
POSTAL SERVICE

U.S. POSTAGE PAID
COSHOCTON, OH
$3.94

How will I know when my Medicare SNF (Skilled Nursing Facility) coverage is ending?

If you are in the <u>Original Medicare Plan</u> and no longer qualify for Medicare coverage, you must be given a written "<u>Notice of Medicare Non-Coverage</u>." The purpose of this notice is to let you know that the SNF believes you no longer qualify for SNF services paid by Medicare. If someone is acting on your behalf, the facility must notify them in writing. Medicare coverage ends the day after you get the notice.

Notice received May 16, 2002

The Notice of <u>Medicare Non-Coverage</u> must tell you:

- The date your Medicare coverage will end (and you must start to pay),

- Why your stay is not (or is no longer) covered,

- Your right to request that the SNF send Medicare its opinion that your care no longer meets Medicare coverage requirements (see page 23).

- That, if you request a Demand Bill (see page 23), you are not required to pay for your SNF stay until you are informed of Medicare's decision* (you do have to pay any coinsurance charged and for services and supplies not covered by Medicare).

- Where you (or someone acting on your behalf) should sign to show you got the notice.

NOTE: If you are in a Medicare Managed Care Plan or a Medicare Private Fee-for-Service Plan, check with your plan to find out how they will let you know your Medicare coverage is ending. You can ask for advance notice of non-coverage from the plan or the SNF. If you don't agree with the decision, you may then file an appeal (see page 23).

* However, you will be responsible for the cost of the stay if Medicare determines you did not meet Medicare criteria.

Words in blue are defined on pages 39-40.

MEDICARE PAYS

Call Palmetto and about this 1-800-282-0530

Services and Supplies	Medicare Pays

Medicare Part A

Hospital Stays During Any One Benefit Period

Days 1 through 60	All but the Part A Inpatient Hospital Deductible amount
Days 61 through 90	All but 25% of the Part A Inpatient Hospital Deductible amount each day
Days 91 and after, when you use Lifetime Reserve Days	All but 50% of the Part A Inpatient Hospital Deductible amount each day
After all Lifetime Reserve Days have been used	Not covered

Blood

1st 3 Pints of Blood or Equivalent Quantities of Packed Red Blood Cells	All but the first 3 pints of blood per calendar year

Skilled Nursing Facility Stays During Any One Benefit Period

Days 1 through 20	100% of the Medicare approved amount
Days 21 through 100	All but 12.5% of the Part A Inpatient Hospital Deductible amount each day

Medicare Part B

Medical Care Each Calendar Year

Medicare Part B Deductible	Not covered
Medical Care Each Calendar Year	80% of the Medicare approved amount after the Medicare Part B Deductible is satisfied

Blood

1st 3 Pints of Blood or Equivalent Quantities of Packed Red Blood Cells	All but the first 3 pints of blood per calendar year.

Additional Services Not Covered By Medicare

Emergency Medical Care In Foreign Countries	At-Home Recovery Care
Outpatient Prescription Drugs	Preventive Medical Care

Newcomerstown, OH 43832

Dec. 26, 2002

Health Care Financing Administration
Department of Health and Human Services
200 Independence Avenue, S.W.
Washington, D.D. 20201

Re: Ralph L. Pollock,
Case Number F14030089   Provider: College Park Nursing and Rehab.
Insurance: Medicare Part A & B; AARP Plan A

Vs: Autumn Healthcare of Coshocton, P.O. Box 727, Coshocton, OH 43812

Responsible Party: Mabel V. Pollock, wife, of 21291 T.R. 287
Newcomerstown, OH 43832. Telephone 740-498-7390

Ralph L. Pollock, an advanced Alzheimer's patient, was a patient in
Coshocton County Memorial Hospital, Coshocton, Ohio from February 4
to February 15, 2002, suffering from stroke, pneumonia and other
conditions. He has been unable to swallow since then and also has
no bowel or bladder control. A gastrostomy tube was installed.

From February 15, 2002 to June 17, 2002, he was a patient in Autumn
Healthcare of Coshocton, Ohio.

On May 16, I received a certified letter from Autumn Healthcare
informing me that, as of May 5, Medicare would no longer pay for
his care. According to the Patient's Rights, I believe the Care
Center was required to notify me in advance of such action.

On June 10, I paid $1,875 which they said would pay the account
until May 5. At that time, because of the expense I began to
make arrangements to take him home. On June 17, I took him home
but, when I found it was too difficult for me to care for him,
on July 8th I placed him in Bell Nursing Home, Kimbolton.

After they began sending me bills which were confusing, I contacted
Medicare and asked that the account be audited.

The charges escalated from $3375. as of 5/13/02, to $7659.68 as of
5/31/02; to $4853.60 as of 7/31/02, then, to 10, 842.10 as of 9/30/02
; to $11,004.73 as of 10/31/02; $11,169.80 as of 11/30/02; $11,337.34
as of 12/31/02; $11,507.40 as of 01/31/03; $11,680.01 as of 02/28/03;
$11,855.21 as of 3/31/03 and $12,213.52 as of 05/31/03. A total of
$1371.42 in interest was included. Some of these bills had a charge
for Jevity, his liquid nutrition, which Medicare will cover.

I contacted Kevin Bartow of CMS who said that it would be investigated
and they could not charge interest as long as it is under investigation.
and they can not charge for Jevity which Medicare will pay.

Mabel V. Pollock, P.O.A. for Ralph L. Pollock, deceased 2/7/03 .

Mabel V. Pollock

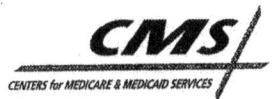

AdminaStar Federal
A CMS Contracted Carrier and Intermediary
http://www.adminastar.com

February 19, 2003

MR. RALPH POLLOCK
21291 TR 257

NEWCOMERSTOWN, OH 43832-0000

RE: Case Number: FI4030089
       Provider: COLLEGE PARK NURSING & REHAB CT *(Autumn Care.)*

Dear MR. POLLOCK:

This is in response to the inquiry we received concerning the above named provider. We will investigate your concerns and let you know the results as soon as the investigation is complete.

We appreciate your interest in eliminating Medicare fraud and want to thank you for bringing this matter to our attention. We want to assure you that this matter will be investigated fully.

Sincerely,

~~Joe Carney~~

~~Joe Carney~~
Analyst
Medicare Benefit Integrity Unit

8115 Knue Road • Indianapolis, IN 46250
Benefit Integrity Unit
Phone: (317) 841-4400   Fax: (317) 841-4600

MAKE CHECK PAYABLE TO

(copy)

AUTUMN HEALTHCARE OF COSHOCTON
P.O. BOX 727
COSHOCTON, OH 43812

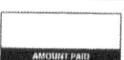

STATEMENT

ACCOUNT NO.	DATE
5419	5/13/02

AMOUNT PAID

NAME
RALPH POLLOCK

MABEL POLLOCK
21291 TR 257
NEWCOMERSTOWN, OH 43832

DETACH AND RETURN THIS PORTION WITH YOUR REMITTANCE

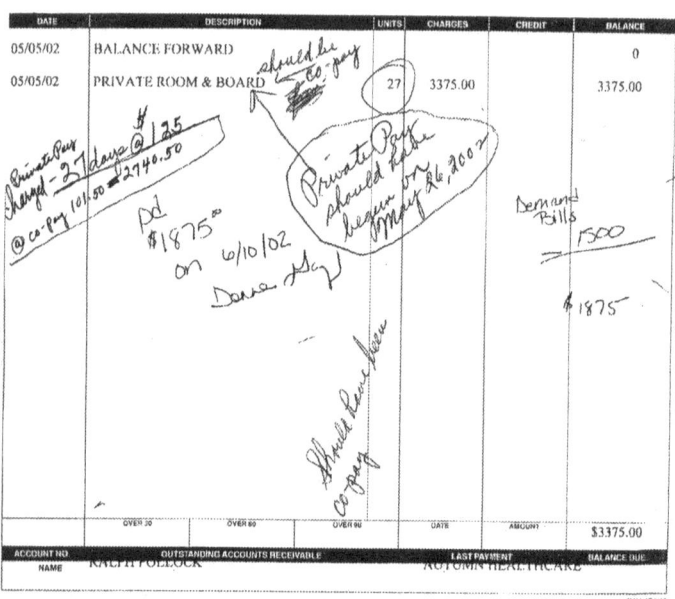

DATE	DESCRIPTION	UNITS	CHARGES	CREDIT	BALANCE
05/05/02	BALANCE FORWARD				0
05/05/02	PRIVATE ROOM & BOARD	27	3375.00		3375.00

	OVER 30	OVER 60	OVER 90	DATE	AMOUNT	
						$3375.00

ACCOUNT NO.	OUTSTANDING ACCOUNTS RECEIVABLE	LAST PAYMENT	BALANCE DUE
NAME	RALPH POLLOCK	AUTUMN HEALTHCARE	

ITEM L/54110

(c o p y)

AUTUMN HEALTHCARE
COSHOCTON
O. BOX 727
COSHOCTON, OH 43812

DON'T FORGET FATHERS DAY IS SUNDAY, JUNE 16TH

MABEL POLLOCK
21291 TR 257

NEWCOMERSTOWN   OH   43832

STATEMENT

ACCOUNT NO.	DATE
	5/31/02

AMOUNT PAID

NAME
RALPH L POLLOCK

DETACH AND RETURN THIS PORTION WITH YOUR REMITTANCE

DATE	DESCRIPTION	UNITS	CHARGES	CREDIT	BALANCE
5/01/02	BALANCE FORWARD—PRIVATE				0.00
5/31/02	PRIVATE NDP R & B	27	3375.00		3375.00
5/01/02	PRIVATE NDP R & B	30	3750.00		7125.00
5/20/02	PRIVATE NDP SUPPLIES	1	534.68		7659.68

Medicare should Pay this!

	OVER 30 0.00	OVER 60 0.00	OVER 90 0.00	DATE	AMOUNT .00	7659.68
COUNT NO.	OUTSTANDING ACCOUNTS RECEIVABLE			LAST PAYMENT		BALANCE DUE
NAME RALPH L POLLOCK			AUTUMN HEALTHCARE			

ITEM OS4836

MAKE CHECK PAYABLE TO

AUTUMN HEALTHCARE
COSHOCTON
P.O. BOX 727
COSHOCTON, OH 43812

STATEMENT

ACCOUNT NO.	DATE
5419	7/31/02

WE APPRECIATE YOUR CONFIDENCE IN US !! THANK YOU.

AMOUNT PAID

MABEL POLLOCK
21291 TR 257

NEWCOMERSTOWN   OH   43832

NAME

RALPH L POLLOCK

DETACH AND RETURN THIS PORTION WITH YOUR REMITTANCE

DATE	DESCRIPTION	UNITS	CHARGES	CREDIT	BALANCE
7/01/02	BALANCE FORWARD—PVT CROSS				4853.60

Notified 5/16/02

60 - day - 101.50 = 1218.00 #

Private Pay should have started May 16,02

5/5 - 5/16/02 - 12 days @ $125.00/ day = $ 1500.00

*These days & this amount of money is not due
to Autumn Health Care until Medicare
makes a determination of coverage.*

*4853.60
-1500.00
$ 3353.60 Due to facility at this time.*

JAddy

Please make payment.

THANK YOU FOR YOUR COOPERATION

5419	OVER 90 818.92	OVER 60 3034.68	OVER 30 0.00	DATE 6/14/02	AMOUNT 1875.00	4853.60

ACCOUNT NO.	OUTSTANDING ACCOUNTS RECEIVABLE	LAST PAYMENT	BALANCE DUE
NAME RALPH L POLLOCK		AUTUMN HEALTHCARE	

ITEM C5#

AUTUMN HEALTHCARE OF COSHOCTON
P.O. BOX 727
COSHOCTON, OH 43812

STATEMENT

ACCOUNT NO.	DATE
	9/30/02

AMOUNT PAID

NAME

MABEL POLLOCK
21291 TR 257
NEWCOMERSTOWN, OH 43832

RALPH POLLOCK

DETACH AND RETURN THIS PORTION WITH YOUR REMITTANCE

DATE	DESCRIPTION	UNITS	CHARGES	CREDIT	BALANCE
	ADMIT 2/15/02 MEDICARE PART A COVERED. MEDICARE PART A COINSURANCE STARTED ON 3/7/02. LAST COVERED MEDICARE PART A DAY WAS 5/4/02. MEDICARE DEMAND BILL IN PROCESS FOR 5/5-5/16/02. TO PRIVATE PAY ON 5/5/02. DISCHARGE 6/17/02				
3/7-3/31/02	MEDICARE PART A COINSURANCE @ $101.50/DAY. INSURANCE WILL NOT PAY.	25	2537.50 ✓		2537.50
4/1-4/30/02	MEDICARE PART A COINSURANCE @ $101.50/DAY. INSURANCE WILL NOT PAY.	30	3045.00		5582.50
5/1-5/4/02	MEDICARE PART A COINSURANCE @ $101.50/DAY. INSURANCE WILL NOT PAY.	4	406.00		5988.50
5/5-5/31/02	PRIVATE PAY ROOM & BOARD @ $125.00/DAY	27	3375.00		9363.50
5/20/02	PRIVATE SUPPLIES		534.68		9898.18
6/1-6/16/02	PRIVATE PAY ROOM & BOARD @ $125.00/DAY	16	2000.00		11,898.18
6/16/02	PRIVATE SUPPLIES		818.92		12,717.10
6/14/02	CASH RECEIPTS-CHECK # 6343			-1875.00	10,842.10
					$10,842.10

	OVER 30	OVER 60	OVER 90	DATE	AMOUNT

ACCOUNT NO.	OUTSTANDING ACCOUNTS RECEIVABLE	LAST PAYMENT	BALANCE DUE
NAME RALPH POLLOCK		AUTUMN HEALTHCARE	

ITEM G841

LEATLAND ■ To Order Call. 800-366-5411

MAKE CHECK PAYABLE TO

AUTUMN HEALTHCARE OF COSHOCTON
P.O. BOX 727
COSHOCTON, OH 43812

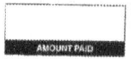

	STATEMENT
ACCOUNT NO.	DATE
	10/31/02

MABEL POLLOCK
21291 TR 257

NEWCOMERSTOWN, OH 43832

AMOUNT PAID
NAME
RALPH POLLOCK

DETACH AND RETURN THIS PORTION WITH YOUR REMITTANCE

DATE	DESCRIPTION	UNITS	CHARGES	CREDIT	BALANCE
10/01/02	BALANCE FORWARD-PRIVATE				10842.10
10/31/02	INTEREST 1.5% ON 10842.10		162.63		11004.73

	OVER 30	OVER 60	10842.10	DATE	AMOUNT	
ACCOUNT NO.	OUTSTANDING ACCOUNTS RECEIVABLE			LAST PAYMENT		BALANCE DUE
NAME	RALPH POLLOCK			AUTUMN HEALTHCARE		

(copy)

AUTUMN HEALTHCARE OF COSHOCTON
P.O. BOX 727
COSHOCTON, OH 43812

STATEMENT

ACCOUNT NO.	DATE
	11/30/02

MABEL POLLOCK
21291 TR 257

NEWCOMERSTOWN, OH 43832

AMOUNT PAID

NAME
RALPH POLLOCK

DETACH AND RETURN THIS PORTION WITH YOUR REMITTANCE

DATE	DESCRIPTION	UNITS	CHARGES	CREDIT	BALANCE
/01/02	BALANCE FORWARD-PRIVATE				11004.73
/30/02	INTEREST 1.5% ON 11004.73		165.07		11169.80

OVER 90	OVER 60	OVER 90	DATE	AMOUNT	11169.80

COUNT NO.	OUTSTANDING ACCOUNTS RECEIVABLE		LAST PAYMENT	BALANCE DUE
NAME	RALPH POLLOCK		AUTUMN HEALTHCARE	

ITEM CS4630F

LAND ● To Order Call. 800-968-5611

MAKE CHECK PAYABLE TO

AUTUMN HEALTHCARE OF COSHOCTON
P.O. BOX 727
COSHOCTON, OH 43812

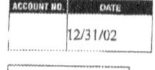

STATEMENT

ACCOUNT NO.	DATE
	12/31/02

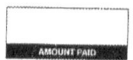

MABEL POLLOCK
21291 TR 257

NEWCOMERSTOWN, OH 43832

AMOUNT PAID	

NAME
RALPH POLLOCK

DETACH AND RETURN THIS PORTION WITH YOUR REMITTANCE

DATE	DESCRIPTION	UNITS	CHARGES	CREDIT	BALANCE
2/01/02	BALANCE FORWARD-PRIVATE				11169.80
2/31/02	INTEREST 1.5% ON 11169.80		167.54		11337.34

	OVER 30	OVER 60	OVER 90	DATE	AMOUNT	11337.34

ACCOUNT NO.	OUTSTANDING ACCOUNTS RECEIVABLE		LAST PAYMENT	BALANCE DUE
NAME	RALPH POLLOCK		AUTUMN HEALTHCARE	

FATLAND ■ To Order Call 800-968-5611

ITEM C?

MAKE CHECK PAYABLE TO

AUTUMN HEALTHCARE OF COSHOCTON
P.O. BOX 727
COSHOCTON, OH 43812

ACCOUNT NO.	DATE
	01/31/03

AMOUNT PAID

MABEL POLLOCK
21291 TR 257
NEWCOMERSTOWN, OH 43832

NAME

RALPH POLLOCK

DETACH AND RETURN THIS PORTION WITH YOUR REMITTANCE

DATE	DESCRIPTION	UNITS	CHARGES	CREDIT	BALANCE
01/01/03	BALANCE FORWARD-PRIVATE				11337.34
01/31/03	INTEREST 1.5% ON 11337.34		1170.06		11507.40

	OVER 70	OVER 80	OVER 90	DATE	AMOUNT	11507.40
ACCOUNT NO.	OUTSTANDING ACCOUNTS RECEIVABLE			LAST PAYMENT		BALANCE DUE
NAME	RALPH POLLOCK			AUTUMN HEALTHCARE		

ITEM C9¢

STLAND ■ To Order Call: 800-988-5511

AUTUMN HEALTHCARE OF COSHOCTON
P.O. BOX 727
COSHOCTON, OH 43812

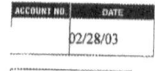

ACCOUNT NO.	DATE
	02/28/03

AMOUNT PAID

MABEL POLLOCK
21291 TR 257
NEWCOMERSTOWN, OH 43832

NAME
RALPH POLLOCK

DETACH AND RETURN THIS PORTION WITH YOUR REMITTANCE

DATE	DESCRIPTION	UNITS	CHARGES	CREDIT	BALANCE
2/01/03	BALANCE FORWARD-PRIVATE				11507.40
2/28/03	INTEREST 1.5%		172.61		11680.01

	OVER 30	OVER 60	OVER 90	DATE	AMOUNT	11680.01
ACCOUNT NO.	OUTSTANDING ACCOUNTS RECEIVABLE			LAST PAYMENT		BALANCE DUE
NAME	RALPH POLLOCK			AUTUMN HEALTHCARE		

ITEM C3

MAKE CHECK PAYABLE TO

AUTUMN HEALTHCARE
COSHOCTON
P.O. BOX 727
OSHOCTON, OH 43812

ACCOUNT NO.	DATE
	3/31/03

MABEL POLLOCK
21291 TR 257

NEWCOMERSTOWN   OH   43832

AMOUNT PAID
NAME
RALPH L POLLOCK

DETACH AND RETURN THIS PORTION WITH YOUR REMITTANCE

DATE	DESCRIPTION	UNITS	CHARGES	CREDIT	BALANCE
3/01/03	BALANCE FORWARD–PRIVATE				11680.01
3/31/03	INTEREST 1.5%		175.20		11855.21

'19	OVER 30 172.61	OVER 60 170.06	OVER 90 11337.34	DATE 6/14/02	AMOUNT 1875.00	11855.21
ACCOUNT NO.	OUTSTANDING ACCOUNTS RECEIVABLE			LAST PAYMENT		BALANCE DUE
NAME RALPH L POLLOCK			AUTUMN HEALTHCARE			

ITEM C848-

JATLAND ■ To Order Call 800-968-5611

AUTUMN HEALTHCARE OF COSHOCTON
P.O. BOX 727
COSHOCTON, OH 43812

ACCOUNT NO.	DATE
	05/31/03

MABEL POLLOCK
21291 TR 257
NEWCOMERSTOWN, OH 43832

AMOUNT PAID

NAME
RALPH POLLOCK

DATE	DESCRIPTION	UNITS	CHARGES	CREDIT	BALANCE
5/01/03	BALANCE FORWARD-PRIVATE				11680.01
3/31/03	INTEREST 1.5%		175.20		11855.21
4/30/03	INTEREST 1.5%		177.82		12033.03
5/31/03	INTEREST 1.5%		180.49		12213.52

18% Interest

	OVER 30	OVER 60	OVER 90	DATE	AMOUNT	
						12213.52

ACCOUNT NO.	OUTSTANDING ACCOUNTS RECEIVABLE	LAST PAYMENT	BALANCE DUE
NAME	RALPH POLLOCK	AUTUMN HEALTHCARE	

ITEM CL.

AUTUMN HEALTHCARE OF COSHOCTON
P.O. BOX 727
COSHOCTON, OH 43812

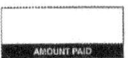

STATEMENT

ACCOUNT NO.	DATE
	06/30/03

MABEL POLLOCK
21291 TR 257
NEWCOMERSTOWN, OH 43832

AMOUNT PAID
NAME
RALPH POLLOCK

DETACH AND RETURN THIS PORTION WITH YOUR REMITTANCE

DATE	DESCRIPTION	UNITS	CHARGES	CREDIT	BALANCE
06/01/03	BALANCE FORWARD-PRIVATE				12213.52
06/30/03	INTEREST 1.5%		183.20		12396.72

*Charged
Total Interest from
10/31/02 to 6/30/03
#1371.42*

	OVER 30	OVER 60	OVER 90	DATE	AMOUNT	12396.72
ACCOUNT NO.	OUTSTANDING ACCOUNTS RECEIVABLE			LAST PAYMENT		BALANCE DUE
NAME	RALPH POLLOCK			AUTUMN HEALTHCARE		

ITEM C84* *

EATLAND ■ To Order Call: 800-968-5611

AUTUMN HEALTHCARE OF COSHOCTON
P.O. BOX 727
COSHOCTON, OH 43812

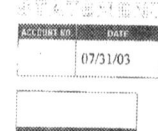

ACCOUNT NO.	DATE
	07/31/03

MABEL POLLOCK
21291 TR 257
NEWCOMERSTOWN, OH 43832

AMOUNT PAID

NAME

RALPH POLLOCK

DETACH AND RETURN THIS PORTION WITH YOUR REMITTANCE

DATE	DESCRIPTION	UNITS	CHARGES	CREDIT	BALANCE
07/01/03	BALANCE FORWARD-PRIVATE				12396.72
07/31/03	INTEREST 1.5%		185.95		12582.67

OVER 30	OVER 60	OVER 90	DATE	AMOUNT	12582.67

ACCOUNT NO.	OUTSTANDING ACCOUNTS RECEIVABLE		LAST PAYMENT	BALANCE DUE
NAME	RALPH POLLOCK		AUTUMN HEALTHCARE	

ITEM C84™

MAKE CHECK PAYABLE TO

AUTUMN HEALTHCARE OF COSHOCTON
P.O. BOX 727
COSHOCTON, OH 43812

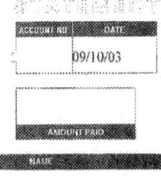

ACCOUNT NO	DATE
	09/10/03

MABEL POLLOCK
21291 TR 257
NEWCOMERSTOWN, OH 43832

AMOUNT PAID

NAME
RALPH POLLOCK

DETACH AND RETURN THIS PORTION WITH YOUR REMITTANCE

DATE	DESCRIPTION	UNITS	CHARGES	CREDIT	BALANCE
08/01/03	BALANCE FORWARD-PRIVATE				12582.67
08/31/03	INTEREST 1.5%		188.74		12771.41

	OVER 30	OVER 60	OVER 90	DATE	AMOUNT	12771.41
ACCOUNT NO	OUTSTANDING ACCOUNTS RECEIVABLE			LAST PAYMENT		BALANCE DUE
NAME	RALPH POLLOCK			AUTUMN HEALTHCARE		

ITEM

GREATLAND ■ To Order Call: 800-968-1611

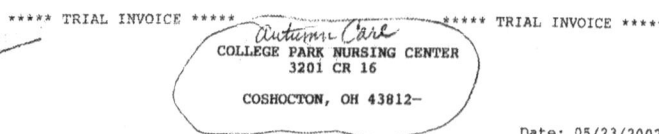

COLLEGE PARK NURSING CENTER
3201 CR 16

COSHOCTON, OH 43812—

Date: 05/23/2002

0 PRIVATE
INVOICE

Page: 1

For Products Used From 04/21/2002 Through 05/20/2002

POLLOCK, RALPH
MABEL POLLOCK
21291 TR 257

NEWCOMERSTOWN, OH 43832—

Patient ID : 5423
Wing   : A
Reference #:
Doctor Name: DR. A. SHAH
Invoice # :

Date	Product #	Description	HCPC	A/R Reference	Qty	Price	Total
Product Family: FS		**– FOOD SUPPLEMENTS**					
05/05/2002	68202600	JEVITY 1000ML RTH			2	10.40	20.80
05/06/2002	68202600	JEVITY 1000ML RTH			2	10.40	20.80
05/07/2002	68202600	JEVITY 1000ML RTH			2	10.40	20.80
05/08/2002	68202600	JEVITY 1000ML RTH			2	10.40	20.80
05/09/2002	68202600	JEVITY 1000ML RTH			2	10.40	20.80
05/10/2002	68202600	JEVITY 1000ML RTH			2	10.40	20.80
05/11/2002	68202600	JEVITY 1000ML RTH			2	10.40	20.80
05/12/2002	68202600	JEVITY 1000ML RTH			2	10.40	20.80
05/13/2002	68202600	JEVITY 1000ML RTH			2	10.40	20.80
05/14/2002	68202600	JEVITY 1000ML RTH			2	10.40	20.80
05/15/2002	68202600	JEVITY 1000ML RTH			2	10.40	20.80
05/16/2002	68202600	JEVITY 1000ML RTH			2	10.40	20.80
05/17/2002	68202600	JEVITY 1000ML RTH			2	10.40	20.80
05/18/2002	68202600	JEVITY 1000ML RTH			2	10.40	20.80
05/19/2002	68202600	JEVITY 1000ML RTH			2	10.40	20.80
05/20/2002	68202600	JEVITY 1000ML RTH			2	10.40	20.80
						Sub-Total:	332.80
Product Family: IN		**– INCONTINENCE**					
05/20/2002	20223100	DRY COMFORT MED			1	7.08	7.08
05/20/2002	20223100	DRY COMFORT MED			1	7.08	7.08
05/20/2002	75053100	PAD CURITY W/ADHES 8#			1	6.76	6.76
						Sub-Total:	20.92
Product Family: MS		**– MED-SURG**					
05/05/2002	38622700	ASPIRIN ENTERIC 81MG 1000			1	0.04	0.04
05/05/2002	88004600	PFS SPIKE COMPANION			1	9.34	9.34
05/05/2002	96651900	SYR IRRG PISTON 60CC			1	1.08	1.08
05/06/2002	38622700	ASPIRIN ENTERIC 81MG 1000			1	0.04	0.04
05/06/2002	88004600	PFS SPIKE COMPANION			1	9.34	9.34
05/06/2002	96651900	SYR IRRG PISTON 60CC			1	1.08	1.08
05/07/2002	38622700	ASPIRIN ENTERIC 81MG 1000			1	0.04	0.04
05/07/2002	88004600	PFS SPIKE COMPANION			1	9.34	9.34
05/07/2002	96651900	SYR IRRG PISTON 60CC			1	1.08	1.08
05/08/2002	38622700	ASPIRIN ENTERIC 81MG 1000			1	0.04	0.04
05/08/2002	88004600	PFS SPIKE COMPANION			1	9.34	9.34
05/08/2002	96651900	SYR IRRG PISTON 60CC			1	1.08	1.08
05/09/2002	38622700	ASPIRIN ENTERIC 81MG 1000			1	0.04	0.04
05/09/2002	88004600	PFS SPIKE COMPANION			1	9.34	9.34
05/09/2002	96651900	SYR IRRG PISTON 60CC			1	1.08	1.08

COLLEGE PARK NURSING CENTER
3201 CR 16

COSHOCTON, OH 43812-

Date: 05/23/2002

0 PRIVATE
INVOICE

Page: 2

For Products Used From 04/21/2002 Through 05/20/2002

POLLOCK, RALPH
MABEL POLLOCK
21291 TR 257

NEWCOMERSTOWN, OH 43832-

Patient ID : 5423
Wing   : A
Reference #:
Doctor Name: DR. A. SHAH
Invoice # :

Date	Product #	Description	HCPC	A/R Reference	Qty	Price	Total
05/10/2002	38622700	ASPIRIN ENTERIC 81MG 1000			1	0.04	0.04
05/10/2002	88004600	PFS SPIKE COMPANION			1	9.34	9.34
05/10/2002	96651900	SYR IRRG PISTON 60CC			1	1.08	1.08
05/11/2002	38622700	ASPIRIN ENTERIC 81MG 1000			1	0.04	0.04
05/11/2002	88004600	PFS SPIKE COMPANION			1	9.34	9.34
05/11/2002	96651900	SYR IRRG PISTON 60CC			1	1.08	1.08
05/12/2002	38622700	ASPIRIN ENTERIC 81MG 1000			1	0.04	0.04
05/12/2002	88004600	PFS SPIKE COMPANION			1	9.34	9.34
05/12/2002	96651900	SYR IRRG PISTON 60CC			1	1.08	1.08
05/13/2002	38622700	ASPIRIN ENTERIC 81MG 1000			1	0.04	0.04
05/13/2002	88004600	PFS SPIKE COMPANION			1	9.34	9.34
05/13/2002	96651900	SYR IRRG PISTON 60CC			1	1.08	1.08
05/14/2002	38622700	ASPIRIN ENTERIC 81MG 1000			1	0.04	0.04
05/14/2002	88004600	PFS SPIKE COMPANION			1	9.34	9.34
05/14/2002	96651900	SYR IRRG PISTON 60CC			1	1.08	1.08
05/15/2002	38622700	ASPIRIN ENTERIC 81MG 1000			1	0.04	0.04
05/15/2002	88004600	PFS SPIKE COMPANION			1	9.34	9.34
05/15/2002	96651900	SYR IRRG PISTON 60CC			1	1.08	1.08
05/16/2002	38622700	ASPIRIN ENTERIC 81MG 1000			1	0.04	0.04
05/16/2002	88004600	PFS SPIKE COMPANION			1	9.34	9.34
05/16/2002	96651900	SYR IRRG PISTON 60CC			1	1.08	1.08
05/17/2002	38622700	ASPIRIN ENTERIC 81MG 1000			1	0.04	0.04
05/17/2002	88004600	PFS SPIKE COMPANION			1	9.34	9.34
05/17/2002	96651900	SYR IRRG PISTON 60CC			1	1.08	1.08
05/18/2002	38622700	ASPIRIN ENTERIC 81MG 1000			1	0.04	0.04
05/18/2002	88004600	PFS SPIKE COMPANION			1	9.34	9.34
05/18/2002	96651900	SYR IRRG PISTON 60CC			1	1.08	1.08
05/19/2002	38622700	ASPIRIN ENTERIC 81MG 1000			1	0.04	0.04
05/19/2002	88004600	PFS SPIKE COMPANION			1	9.34	9.34
05/19/2002	96651900	SYR IRRG PISTON 60CC			1	1.08	1.08
05/20/2002	23742000	SPONGE SOF-WICK 2X2 6PLY			1	0.34	1.02
05/20/2002	23742000	SPONGE SOF-WICK 2X2 6PLY			1	0.34	0.34
05/20/2002	23922000	SPONG IV SOF-WICK 2X2"6PL			3	0.50	1.50
05/20/2002	23922000	SPONG IV SOF-WICK 2X2"6PL			9	0.50	4.50
05/20/2002	23922000	SPONG IV SOF-WICK 2X2"6PL			2	0.50	1.00
05/20/2002	38622700	ASPIRIN ENTERIC 81MG 1000			1	0.04	0.04
05/20/2002	66862100	OPSITE + DRSG COMP 2X2			1	0.60	0.60
05/20/2002	88004600	PFS SPIKE COMPANION			1	9.34	9.34
05/20/2002	93301700	SHAVING CREAM 11OZ			1	2.32	2.32
05/20/2002	93301700	SHAVING CREAM 11OZ			1	2.32	2.32
05/20/2002	96651900	SYR IRRG PISTON 60CC			1	1.08	1.08

COLLEGE PARK NURSING CENTER
3201 CR 16

COSHOCTON, OH 43812—

Date: 05/23/2002

0 PRIVATE
INVOICE

Page: 3

For Products Used From 04/21/2002 Through 05/20/2002

POLLOCK, RALPH   Patient ID : 5423
MABEL POLLOCK   Wing   : A
21291 TR 257   Reference #:
                                  Doctor Name: DR. A. SHAH
NEWCOMERSTOWN, OH 43832—   Invoice # :

Date	Product #	Description	HCPC	A/R Reference	Qty	Price	Total

Sub-Total: 180.96

***** THIS IS A TRIAL INVOICE *****

Total Amount Due: 534.68

AUTUMN HEALTH CARE
3201 CR 16

COSHOCTON, OH 43812-

Date: 06/24/2002

0 PRIVATE
INVOICE

Page: 1

For Products Used From 05/21/2002 Through 06/20/2002

POLLOCK, RALPH
MABEL POLLOCK
21291 TR 257

NEWCOMERSTOWN, OH 43832-

Patient ID : 5423
Wing   : A
Reference #:
Doctor Name: DR. A. SHAH
Invoice # :

Date	Product #	Description	HCPC	A/R Reference	Qty	Price	Total
Product Family: FS		**- FOOD SUPPLEMENTS**					
05/21/2002	68202600	JEVITY 1000ML RTH			2	10.40	20.80
05/22/2002	68202600	JEVITY 1000ML RTH			2	10.40	20.80
05/23/2002	68202600	JEVITY 1000ML RTH			2	10.40	20.80
05/24/2002	68202600	JEVITY 1000ML RTH			2	10.40	20.80
05/25/2002	68202600	JEVITY 1000ML RTH			2	10.40	20.80
05/26/2002	68202600	JEVITY 1000ML RTH			2	10.40	20.80
05/27/2002	68202600	JEVITY 1000ML RTH			2	10.40	20.80
05/28/2002	68202600	JEVITY 1000ML RTH			2	10.40	20.80
05/29/2002	68202600	JEVITY 1000ML RTH			2	10.40	20.80
05/30/2002	68202600	JEVITY 1000ML RTH			2	10.40	20.80
05/31/2002	68202600	JEVITY 1000ML RTH			2	10.40	20.80
06/01/2002	68202600	JEVITY 1000ML RTH			2	10.40	20.80
06/02/2002	68202600	JEVITY 1000ML RTH			2	10.40	20.80
06/03/2002	68202600	JEVITY 1000ML RTH			2	10.40	20.80
06/04/2002	68202600	JEVITY 1000ML RTH			2	10.40	20.80
06/05/2002	31282600	JEVITY + 8OZ CAN			8	2.72	21.76
06/06/2002	31282600	JEVITY + 8OZ CAN			8	2.72	21.76
06/07/2002	31282600	JEVITY + 8OZ CAN			8	2.72	21.76
06/08/2002	31282600	JEVITY + 8OZ CAN			8	2.72	21.76
06/09/2002	31282600	JEVITY + 8OZ CAN			8	2.72	21.76
06/10/2002	31282600	JEVITY + 8OZ CAN			8	2.72	21.76
06/11/2002	31282600	JEVITY + 8OZ CAN			8	2.72	21.76
06/12/2002	31282600	JEVITY + 8OZ CAN			8	2.72	21.76
06/13/2002	31282600	JEVITY + 8OZ CAN			8	2.72	21.76
06/14/2002	31282600	JEVITY + 8OZ CAN			8	2.72	21.76
06/15/2002	31282600	JEVITY + 8OZ CAN			8	2.72	21.76
06/16/2002	31282600	JEVITY + 8OZ CAN			8	2.72	21.76
06/17/2002	31282600	JEVITY + 8OZ CAN			8	2.72	21.76
						Sub-Total:	594.08
Product Family: IN		**- INCONTINENCE**					
06/16/2002	20223100	DRY COMFORT MED			1	7.08	7.08
06/16/2002	30903100	BRIEF DRY COMF EXTRA LG			3	9.42	28.26
						Sub-Total:	35.34
Product Family: MS		**- MED-SURG**					
05/21/2002	38622700	ASPIRIN ENTERIC 81MG 1000			1	0.04	0.04
05/21/2002	88004600	PFS SPIKE COMPANION			1	9.34	9.34
05/21/2002	96651900	SYR IRRG PISTON 60CC			1	1.08	1.08
05/22/2002	38622700	ASPIRIN ENTERIC 81MG 1000			1	0.04	0.04

AUTUMN HEALTH CARE
3201 CR 16

COSHOCTON, OH 43812—

Date: 06/24/2002

0 PRIVATE
INVOICE

Page: 2

For Products Used From 05/21/2002 Through 06/20/2002

POLLOCK, RALPH   Patient ID : 5423
MABEL POLLOCK   Wing   : A
21291 TR 257   Reference #:
                       Doctor Name: DR. A. SHAH
NEWCOMERSTOWN, OH 43832—   Invoice # :

Date	Product #	Description	HCPC	A/R Reference	Qty	Price	Total
05/22/2002	88004600	PFS SPIKE COMPANION			1	9.34	9.34
05/22/2002	96651900	SYR IRRG PISTON 60CC			1	1.08	1.08
05/23/2002	38622700	ASPIRIN ENTERIC 81MG 1000			1	0.04	0.04
05/23/2002	88004600	PFS SPIKE COMPANION			1	9.34	9.34
05/23/2002	96651900	SYR IRRG PISTON 60CC			1	1.08	1.08
05/24/2002	38622700	ASPIRIN ENTERIC 81MG 1000			1	0.04	0.04
05/24/2002	88004600	PFS SPIKE COMPANION			1	9.34	9.34
05/24/2002	96651900	SYR IRRG PISTON 60CC			1	1.08	1.08
05/25/2002	38622700	ASPIRIN ENTERIC 81MG 1000			1	0.04	0.04
05/25/2002	88004600	PFS SPIKE COMPANION			1	9.34	9.34
05/25/2002	96651900	SYR IRRG PISTON 60CC			1	1.08	1.08
05/26/2002	38622700	ASPIRIN ENTERIC 81MG 1000			1	0.04	0.04
05/26/2002	88004600	PFS SPIKE COMPANION			1	9.34	9.34
05/26/2002	96651900	SYR IRRG PISTON 60CC			1	1.08	1.08
05/27/2002	38622700	ASPIRIN ENTERIC 81MG 1000			1	0.04	0.04
05/27/2002	88004600	PFS SPIKE COMPANION			1	9.34	9.34
05/27/2002	96651900	SYR IRRG PISTON 60CC			1	1.08	1.08
05/28/2002	38622700	ASPIRIN ENTERIC 81MG 1000			1	0.04	0.04
05/28/2002	88004600	PFS SPIKE COMPANION			1	9.34	9.34
05/28/2002	96651900	SYR IRRG PISTON 60CC			1	1.08	1.08
05/29/2002	38622700	ASPIRIN ENTERIC 81MG 1000			1	0.04	0.04
05/29/2002	88004600	PFS SPIKE COMPANION			1	9.34	9.34
05/29/2002	96651900	SYR IRRG PISTON 60CC			1	1.08	1.08
05/30/2002	38622700	ASPIRIN ENTERIC 81MG 1000			1	0.04	0.04
05/30/2002	88004600	PFS SPIKE COMPANION			1	9.34	9.34
05/30/2002	96651900	SYR IRRG PISTON 60CC			1	1.08	1.08
05/31/2002	38622700	ASPIRIN ENTERIC 81MG 1000			1	0.04	0.04
05/31/2002	88004600	PFS SPIKE COMPANION			1	9.34	9.34
05/31/2002	96651900	SYR IRRG PISTON 60CC			1	1.08	1.08
06/01/2002	38622700	ASPIRIN ENTERIC 81MG 1000			1	0.04	0.04
06/01/2002	88004600	PFS SPIKE COMPANION			1	9.34	9.34
06/01/2002	96651900	SYR IRRG PISTON 60CC			1	1.08	1.08
06/02/2002	38622700	ASPIRIN ENTERIC 81MG 1000			1	0.04	0.04
06/02/2002	88004600	PFS SPIKE COMPANION			1	9.34	9.34
06/02/2002	96651900	SYR IRRG PISTON 60CC			1	1.08	1.08
06/03/2002	38622700	ASPIRIN ENTERIC 81MG 1000			1	0.04	0.04
06/03/2002	88004600	PFS SPIKE COMPANION			1	9.34	9.34
06/03/2002	96651900	SYR IRRG PISTON 60CC			1	1.08	1.08
06/04/2002	38622700	ASPIRIN ENTERIC 81MG 1000			1	0.04	0.04
06/04/2002	88004600	PFS SPIKE COMPANION			1	9.34	9.34
06/04/2002	96651900	SYR IRRG PISTON 60CC			1	1.08	1.08

AUTUMN HEALTH CARE
3201 CR 16

COSHOCTON, OH 43812-

Date: 06/24/2002

0 PRIVATE
INVOICE

Page: 3

For Products Used From 05/21/2002 Through 06/20/2002

POLLOCK, RALPH
MABEL POLLOCK
21291 TR 257

NEWCOMERSTOWN, OH 43832-

Patient ID : 5423
Wing   : A
Reference #:
Doctor Name: DR. A. SHAH
Invoice # :

Date	Product #	Description	HCPC	A/R Reference	Qty	Price	Total
06/05/2002	38622700	ASPIRIN ENTERIC 81MG 1000			1	0.04	0.04
06/05/2002	96651900	SYR IRRG PISTON 60CC			1	1.08	1.08
06/06/2002	38622700	ASPIRIN ENTERIC 81MG 1000			1	0.04	0.04
06/06/2002	96651900	SYR IRRG PISTON 60CC			1	1.08	1.08
06/07/2002	38622700	ASPIRIN ENTERIC 81MG 1000			1	0.04	0.04
06/07/2002	96651900	SYR IRRG PISTON 60CC			1	1.09	1.08
06/08/2002	38622700	ASPIRIN ENTERIC 81MG 1000			1	0.04	0.04
06/08/2002	96651900	SYR IRRG PISTON 60CC			1	1.08	1.08
06/09/2002	38622700	ASPIRIN ENTERIC 81MG 1000			1	0.04	0.04
06/09/2002	96651900	SYR IRRG PISTON 60CC			1	1.08	1.08
06/10/2002	38622700	ASPIRIN ENTERIC 81MG 1000			1	0.04	0.04
06/10/2002	96651900	SYR IRRG PISTON 60CC			1	1.08	1.08
06/11/2002	38622700	ASPIRIN ENTERIC 81MG 1000			1	0.04	0.04
06/11/2002	96651900	SYR IRRG PISTON 60CC			1	1.08	1.08
06/12/2002	38622700	ASPIRIN ENTERIC 81MG 1000			1	0.04	0.04
06/12/2002	96651900	SYR IRRG PISTON 60CC			1	1.08	1.08
06/13/2002	38622700	ASPIRIN ENTERIC 81MG 1000			1	0.04	0.04
06/13/2002	96651900	SYR IRRG PISTON 60CC			1	1.08	1.08
06/14/2002	38622700	ASPIRIN ENTERIC 81MG 1000			1	0.04	0.04
06/14/2002	96651900	SYR IRRG PISTON 60CC			1	1.08	1.08
06/15/2002	38622700	ASPIRIN ENTERIC 81MG 1000			1	0.04	0.04
06/15/2002	96651900	SYR IRRG PISTON 60CC			1	1.08	1.08
06/16/2002	23742000	SPONGE SOF-WICK 2X2 6PLY			10	0.34	3.40
06/16/2002	23922000	SPONG IV SOF-WICK 2X2 6PL			10	0.50	5.00
06/16/2002	30521800	SHAMP/BWASH AVRA CARE 8OZ			1	2.52	2.52
06/16/2002	38622700	ASPIRIN ENTERIC 81MG 1000			1	0.04	0.04
06/16/2002	93301700	SHAVING CREAM 11OZ			1	2.32	2.32
06/16/2002	96651900	SYR IRRG PISTON 60CC			1	1.08	1.08
06/17/2002	38622700	ASPIRIN ENTERIC 81MG 1000			1	0.04	0.04
06/17/2002	96651900	SYR IRRG PISTON 60CC			1	1.08	1.08

Sub-Total: 188.70

***** THIS IS A TRIAL INVOICE *****

Total Amount Due: 818.92

About the Author

Mabel (Hayes) Pollock was born in North Carolina and moved to Ohio at the age of three. She worked for Civil Service at Dayton during World War II. She later completed courses in fiction and article writing from Writer's Digest School of Cincinnati. She served as a news reporter for The Times Reporter of New Philadelphia; was affiliated with Buckeye Country Magazine of Uhrichsville; did freelancing; and served on the committee to help write the Coshocton County History book which was published in 1985.

In 1943, she married Ralph Pollock who passed away in February, 2003 after suffering from Alzheimer's disease for approximately eight years. She lives on a farm near Newcomers town and has two daughters and four grandchildren.

In addition to THE HEARTBREAK OF ALZHEIMER'S, Mabel is the author of OUR STATE OHIO, published in 2001 and THE CRUSADE OF THE CHILDREN, published in 2002.

www.ingramcontent.com/pod-product-compliance
Lightning Source LLC
Chambersburg PA
CBHW052245290526
45785CB00016B/1306